I0224016

BREAKING
THE
~~YOLK~~
YOKE

BREAKING THE ~~YOLK~~ YOKE

The Biblical Beginning...and End
to Our Struggle With Food

TONI PERRY

GRACE
PUBLISHING
BROKEN ARROW, OK

Unless otherwise indicated, Scripture quotations in this book are taken from *The Study Bible, New International Version.* ©1986, 1992, 1996 by The Zondervan Corporation, and from the *New International Version* online. Used by permission.

Scripture quotations marked KJV are taken from the *King James Version* of the *Bible*.

Scripture quotations marked NASB are taken from the New American Standard Bible, © 1960, 1977 by The Lockman Foundation.

With the exception of brief quotations embodied in a review, this book, or parts thereof may not be reproduced in any form without permission. Photocopying, scanning, uploading, and/or distribution of this book via the Internet or any other means without written permission of the publisher is illegal and punishable by law.

For Information Contact
Grace Publishing
PO Box 1233
Broken Arrow, OK 74013

Cover Design: Kim Althausen

ISBN 13: 978-1-60495-004-5
ISBN 10: 1-60495-004-8

Copyright © 2013 by Toni Perry. Published by Grace Publishing, Broken Arrow, OK. All rights reserved.

About Copyrights

First Timothy 5:17-18 instructs us to give the laborer his wages, specifically those who labor in the Word and doctrine. Even so, some people who would never shoplift may think nothing of copying a book. The results are the same; it's theft.

As Christians, we have a moral, as well as a legal, responsibility to see that authors receive fair compensation for their efforts. Many of them depend on the income from the sale of their books as their livelihood, as do the artists, editors, and numerous other people who work to make their books available to you.

With the exception of brief quotations embodied in a review, this book, or parts thereof may not be reproduced in any form without permission. It is protected by copyright and is not intended to be shared with or duplicated by others who have not purchased it for themselves from authorized sellers. Photocopying, scanning, uploading, and/or distribution of this book via the Internet or any other means without written permission of the publisher is illegal and punishable by law.

If you have a copy of this book that was not purchased by or for you, please be aware that you are using an illegal, pirated copy. Please purchase only authorized editions, from authorized sellers, and do not participate in or encourage piracy of copyrighted materials.

Your support of the author's rights is appreciated.

DEDICATION

To Almighty God

Father, Son, and Holy Spirit

Smile on me, your servant; teach me the right way to live.

Psalm 119:135

and

To George LeGrande Perry

My God-Fearing Husband and Million-Dollar Gold Piece.

My beloved is mine, and I am his . . . .

Song of Solomon 2:16

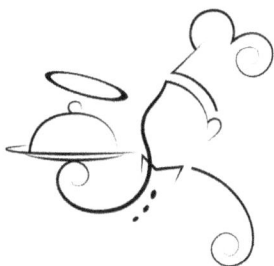

Acknowledgments

With heartfelt thanks, love, and appreciation to the following:

My Lord and Savior, Jesus Christ, for calling me to this unique ministry.

My husband, George, and our beautiful blended family: Adam, Elizabeth, Rebecca, and Natasha; our daughter-in-law, Meghan, and our two granddaughters: Lilliana and Cheyla. Last but not least, all the Perry pets: Isabella, Stinky, Oreo, Jack and Ollie. I prayed to God for a big family and now *my cup runneth over*. (Psalm 23:5)

Sherri McDonald, Director of Women's Ministries at Grace Church in Netcong, New Jersey. Your trust and support enabled me to start on the path toward publication.

Terri Kalfas, Grace Publishing. Three years of waiting for God's timing was rewarded with the desire of my heart — to collaborate with you on this project and share in this ministry.

Karen Moore, author. For your support of this study *from the beginning* and for your contract-reviewing expertise over the years. You kept me from stumbling, and I am forever grateful.

Wayne Martelli, friend and editorial guru. For giving so freely of your time to review materials with me. Lord willing, may there be many more Panera editing sessions in our future.

Roberta Dillis, author of the future children's series *Portage Point Pals*. A predestined, first-timers meeting at the Blue Ridge Mountains Christian Writers Conference

(BRMCWC) in North Carolina blossomed into an incredible friendship. Keeping you lifted in prayer as we go forward in faith.

Dr. Alton Gansky, Edie Melson, Eva Marie Everson, and the rest of the faculty at the BRMCWC who are committed to educating and encouraging aspiring Christian writers.

Kim Althausen, graphic designer. For applying your God-given creativity and talents to this ministry — I am blessed even more because of it.

The God's Kitchen Ministries family: Barbara Guidetti, Cindy Bochniak, Doreen Fusco, Sherri Leonard, Shelli Mance, Ann Marie Gleason, Kathy Rizzo, Alicia Harris, and Jennifer McCord. Inexpressible thanks, ladies.

Julie Tatchell, my British Sister in Christ. Distance can never diminish a friendship that "bears" fruit for Christ!

Pam Terebecke, Soul Sister. You are dearly loved, prayed for, and treasured.

My mother, Jean Angelo. For all your love and prayers, and for giving me my first Bible.

My grandmother, Josephine LoBue (June 9, 1920 – November 28, 1999). An incredible woman who walked with the Lord and taught me the true meaning of food, fellowship, and how to care for others.

Table of Contents

Introduction 11

Lesson 1: Two Gardens 17

    Mise en Place 28

    Forbidden Apple, Walnut and Blue Cheese Salad with Raspberry Vinaigrette 30

Lesson 2: What's Your Beef? 33

    Mise en Place 44

    Noah's Tender Cow Carne on a Raft 46

Lesson 3: Entertaining Angels — Pursuing Hospitality 49

    Mise en Place 56

    Divine Pumpkin Streusel Bread 60

Lesson 4: Out-of-Control Appetites 63

    Mise en Place 70

    Esau's Legacy Lentil Stew 72

Lesson 5: Multi-Colored Temptations (First Course) 75

    Mise en Place 86

    Egyptian Pistachio Couscous with Roasted Chicken 94

Lesson 6: Multi-Colored Temptations (Second Course) 97

    Mise en Place 104

    Pharoah's Fat and Lean Black and White All-Purpose Cake 112

Lesson 7: Multi-Colored Temptations (Third Course) 115

    Mise en Place 126

    Finally Free-keh Pilaf 134

Closing: The Third Garden 137

In Memoriam 140

    Mariann's Homespun & Wholesome Rice Pudding 141

Author Bio 142

Endnotes 143

For all recipes contained in this study, God's Kitchen Ministries encourages the use of Certified Organic/Raw foods to maximize nutrition and gain the most health benefits.

Visit www.Gods-Kitchen.org for photos, and complete nutritional information on each recipe.

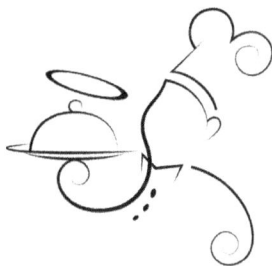

INTRODUCTION

Do not destroy the work of God for the sake of food . . .

Romans 14:20

IN THE BEGINNING, God created the Heavens and the Earth . . .

And He populated the Earth with fruits and vegetables of all kinds — such as broccoli, potatoes, tomatoes, cauliflower, spinach, and multi-colored bell peppers — so that the Man and the Woman would live long, healthy lives.

God said to His newlyweds, "Behold. Try my fresh green salad!"

Then using God's great gifts . . . Satan made processed salad dressing, artificial bacon bits, and Texas-sized garlic toast on the side.

The Man and the Woman ate, gained a pound or two, and Satan smiled.

Then God created wheat to make bread, bees to make honey, and cows to give milk. And Satan fashioned bleached white flour from the wheat and sugar from the cane, then combined them and created cream-filled donuts and triple-decker ice cream sundaes.

And Satan said, "You want chocolate with that?" And Woman said, "Absolutely! As long as you're at it, add some sprinkles."

And the Man and Woman's fig leaves did not fit anymore.

So God said . . . "I have sent you heart-healthy olive oil to use in your salad and with which to cook." And Satan brought forth deep-fried fish and chicken-fried steak.

And Man's cholesterol went through the roof.

God then created running shoes so that His children might enjoy His creation.

And Satan gave Cable TV with a remote control so Man would not have to toil to change channels.

Then Man and Woman laughed and cried before the light of TV . . . and began wearing sweat pants.

So God gave Man lean beef to go with the potato, which was naturally low in fat and brimming with nutrition, so that Man might consume fewer calories and still satisfy his appetite.

And Satan created the 99-cent double cheeseburger. Then Satan said, "You want fries with that?" And Man said, "Yes, and Super-Size them!"

Then Man went into cardiac arrest and Satan said, "It is good."

God sighed and created Quadruple Bypass Surgery.

Then Satan created Health Insurance

The End.[1]

Amusing, yes? The author of this food-related parody on creation is unknown, but the tongue-in-cheek description of Satan's tactics against humanity rings true. This fallen angel and ringleader of demons works very hard at corrupting our healthy desires. He loathes seeing our appetites satisfied and wants us to lust after a good thing until the impulse becomes our master. Reduced to a slave, we are yoked to that desire which — in the proper context — the Lord intended to be freely enjoyed.

"What!" you say. *"Enjoy food freely?"*

Yes, you read correctly. The Lord intended for you and me to have an intimate relationship with Him *and* freely enjoy the food He created — without struggle and without guilt.

So when and where did it all go wrong? The beginning of our struggle with food can be found in the Bible — in the Book of Genesis, Chapter 3 . . . in the Garden of Eden.

Almighty God gave Mr. and Mrs. Mankind a free food supply that spanned the face of the entire earth. It included every seed-bearing plant and tree that has fruit with seed in it. So God made all kinds of trees grow out of the ground — trees pleasing to the eye and good for food. But in the middle of the Garden of Eden stood one tree — just one tree — that the Lord commanded was taboo: the tree of the knowledge of good and evil.

Spurred on by the lies of the serpent, Eve, *the mother of all the living*,[2] began to look at that one tree and its fruit differently. She found the fruit of that tabooed tree pleasing to the eye and good for food, but then she reasoned, from what the serpent had said, that God was cheating her and her husband out of something good . . . something better.

Just one bite was all it took to allow sin and evil to enter the human heart and banish mankind from God's holy presence.

Just one bite was all it took for our sacred hearts, bodies, minds, souls, and spirits to be corrupted.

Just one bite was all it took to ruin our holy relationship with God and all of His creation . . . including a pure and unadulterated connection with food!

So here we are, millennia later, still looking for the solution to the struggle that began with **just one bite**.

In today's culture, Almighty Food has become the new American idol. Food has taken center stage — on cooking shows, talk shows, in magazines, social media blogs, and of course, at our own tables. God's intentional blessing to our bodies and nourishment to our spirits has, instead, become a life-long curse for many of us.

So what is this fascination — this obsession — that caused the first woman to stumble and fall, and many women today to stumble and fall . . . into a vicious love-to-eat / hate-to-eat cycle?

From my earliest memories, my unbalanced eating habits led to constant weight gain and various health issues. During adolescence, I realized I could not meet the image or model-thin body type exemplified in the media trends of the time, a body image which has gained momentum in our contemporary culture.

As a full-figured teenager, I tried to fit in by starving myself so I could wear the latest designer jeans. I recall exasperated efforts of lying flat on the floor, straight-legged, as I worked tight denim over my hips and then attempted to pull and stretch the button across a bulging waistline.

What this experience — and the media — did to my self-esteem started me on a lifelong journey of yo-yo dieting. Yo-yo dieting is "the practice of repeatedly losing weight by dieting, and subsequently regaining it."[3] In simple terms, the dieter is initially successful in the pursuit of weight loss, but unsuccessful in maintaining the weight loss long-term. The dieter then seeks to lose the regained weight, and the cycle begins again.

In my years living on this terra firma, I have tried almost every diet fad and trend on the market, to no avail. My fervent prayers and petitions to God went hand-in-hand with my own efforts to break free from the yoke, the control, and the enslavement of certain foods, eating habits, behaviors, and attitudes.

In 2001 I accepted Jesus Christ as my personal savior, and I earnestly hoped that in addition to the salvation of my soul, He would rescue me from my self-destructive binges and dieting tendencies. I did not realize that His rescue offered so much more. Although my eternal salvation was sealed forever — without my surrender to His lordship, it did not guarantee a godly or fruitful life here on earth.

Our Father's will for us is to live under the lordship of His Son. That means we must submit to Jesus as the one in charge of our life. When we do, Christ provides us with wisdom and direction. (And even though I often make mistakes, He always reminds me that His grace is for imperfect people like you and me.)

After years of studying and teaching His Word, I realized the way I care for my body affects my relationship with God and with others. Committed prayer time on a daily basis showed me that I had not given God complete dominion over my entire life. I had just given him certain areas . . . such as my health issues, family, and career.

So, I pondered and prayed: Does the Bible — the infallible Word of God — have anything to say on the subject of food and eating? Is it truly possible to submit myself to the Lord in this area for permanent transformation?

My path to freedom began with Romans 14:20: *Do not destroy the work of God for the sake of food.* Destroy the work of God. Did He mean . . . me? Was I destroying the work of God with what I ate? A still, small voice whispered the answer: Yes.

So I surrendered my heart, and He brought me deeper into His Word, but with new, unveiled eyes. Eventually, studying God's *truth* about food set me free.

Free from its yoke. Free from its bondage. Free from its tyranny.

Free to fight through the power of Christ Jesus, and with the knowledge of how to win the battle with the sword of the Spirit (which Ephesians 6:17 declares is *the word of God)* hidden in my heart.

King David said it best: *"I have hidden your word in my heart that I might not sin against you"* (Psalm 19:14).

Do you feel as though your body and spirit are at war when it comes to what and how you eat? Tell me, what would happen if you turned to Christ, instead of the fridge, to save you from your troubles?

You can step out of Hell's Kitchen and follow the blessed, fragrant aromas of hope that lead to God's Kitchen.

But, what is God's Kitchen?

With hundreds of references in the Bible, God has revealed how He wants you to eat and what your approach toward eating should be.

This *food and faith* Bible study will empower you to understand God's Word on the subject, and will strengthen your commitment to eat healthy, eat holy, and find comfort in God's provisions.

What distinguishes the God's Kitchen series from other publications, programs, and Bible studies is that this is *not* a diet or a Bible-foods-only plan, but an in-depth study of Scripture as it pertains to food, eating habits, attitudes, and our relationships with Almighty God and others. Throughout this study of Genesis, we will learn life-changing lessons from a few of God's first families, such as Adam and Eve, Noah, Jacob and Esau, Abraham, Isaac, Jacob, and Joseph.

This unique interactive series offers you Christ-centered guidelines for physical and spiritual sustenance. Each lesson includes a food-focused Bible study segment with commentary and a daily devotional. As a tasty bonus, at the end of each lesson, God's Kitchen comes alive with an easy, yet delectable recipe inspired by the people and events in the Book of Genesis — a recipe designed for you to enjoy in your home or with your study group.

So get ready to embark on an incredible, unique journey that can change the course of your life! The Lord, Himself, says:

> *"Why spend money on what is not bread, and your labor on what does not satisfy? Listen, listen to me, and eat what is good, and your soul will delight in the richest of fare."*

Isaiah 55:2

Taste and see how devouring Holy Scripture can help you trust God in all things . . . including your daily bread!

In His Eternal Grip,

Toni Perry

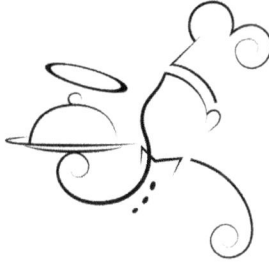

Two Gardens

Our journey begins in two gardens prominently mentioned in the Bible: The Garden of Eden and The Garden of Gethsemane.

Entry is free: The only requirement to pass through these garden gates is to prayerfully open your heart to what God has to say, and then, one day at a time, put into practice what you learn. Second Timothy 2:15 tells us *all Scripture is God-breathed and is useful for teaching, rebuking, correcting and training in righteousness.* If you set your goal to persevere over the next several weeks, you will be amazed at the change in your mental, physical, and spiritual life. If you do not let truth go in one ear and out the other, studying God's Word will change your thinking and your actions. So, let's begin with prayer:

> Heavenly Father, I come to You for help because You are God and nothing is too difficult or even impossible for You. I know it is important to understand Your ways of eating.

> Father, I need Your wisdom, encouragement, strength, and direction. I need confidence to face this life with all its challenges, and I recognize it can only come from You as a gift of grace. Please grant this to me.

> As I study Your Word, meet with me in a personal and intimate way that will equip and sustain me for all that the future holds, in ways that will rebuke and restrain me if I am going the wrong way. My desire, Lord, is to please You. If I am not on the right path, turn me around through Your Word and by Your Holy Spirit. I commit to give this study my all. I ask You to change my life as I

choose the one thing which can never be taken away from me — to sit at Your feet and learn from You. In faith, I thank You for what You are going to do, and pray this in the name of my Lord and King, Jesus Christ, Amen.

Make Up Your Mind

Let's read from Genesis, Chapters 2 and 3.

Chapter 2

Thus the heavens and the earth were completed in all their vast array.

By the seventh day God had finished the work he had been doing; so on the seventh day he rested from all his work. Then God blessed the seventh day and made it holy, because on it he rested from all the work of creating that he had done.

Adam and Eve

This is the account of the heavens and the earth when they were created, when the LORD God made the earth and the heavens.

Now no shrub had yet appeared on the earth and no plant had yet sprung up, for the LORD God had not sent rain on the earth and there was no one to work the ground, but streams came up from the earth and watered the whole surface of the ground. Then the LORD God formed a man from the dust of the ground and breathed into his nostrils the breath of life, and the man became a living being.

Now the LORD God had planted a garden in the east, in Eden; and there he put the man he had formed. The LORD God made all kinds of trees grow out of the ground — trees that were pleasing to the eye and good for food. In the middle of the garden were the tree of life and the tree of the knowledge of good and evil. . . .

The LORD God took the man and put him in the Garden of Eden to work it and take care of it. And the LORD God commanded the man, "You are free to eat from any tree in the garden; but you must not eat from the tree of the knowledge of good and evil, for when you eat from it you will certainly die."

The LORD God said, "It is not good for the man to be alone. I will make a helper suitable for him."

Now the LORD God had formed out of the ground all the wild animals and all the birds in the sky. He brought them to the man to see what he would name them. . . .

But for Adam no suitable helper was found. . . . Then the LORD God made a woman. . . and he brought her to the man. . . .

Adam and his wife were both naked, and they felt no shame.

Chapter 3

The Fall

Now the serpent was more crafty than any of the wild animals the LORD God had made. He said to the woman, "Did God really say, 'You must not eat from any tree in the garden'?"

The woman said to the serpent, "We may eat fruit from the trees in the garden, but God did say, 'You must not eat fruit from the tree that is in the middle of the garden, and you must not touch it, or you will die.'"

"You will not certainly die," the serpent said to the woman. "For God knows that when you eat from it your eyes will be opened, and you will be like God, knowing good and evil."

When the woman saw that the fruit of the tree was good for food and pleasing to the eye, and also desirable for gaining wisdom, she took some and ate it. She also gave some to her husband, who was with her, and he ate it. Then the eyes of both of them were opened, and they realized they were naked; so they sewed fig leaves together and made coverings for themselves.

Then the man and his wife heard the sound of the LORD God as he was walking in the garden in the cool of the day, and they hid from the LORD God among the trees of the garden. ⁹ But the LORD God called to the man, "Where are you?"

He answered, "I heard you in the garden, and I was afraid because I was naked; so I hid."

And he said, "Who told you that you were naked? Have you eaten from the tree that I commanded you not to eat from?"

The man said, "The woman you put here with me — she gave me some fruit from the tree, and I ate it."

Then the LORD God said to the woman, "What is this you have done?"

The woman said, "The serpent deceived me, and I ate.". . .

To Adam he said, "Because you listened to your wife and ate fruit from the tree about which I commanded you, 'You must not eat from it,'

Cursed is the ground because of you;
through painful toil you will eat food from it
all the days of your life.

It will produce thorns and thistles for you,
and you will eat the plants of the field.

By the sweat of your brow
you will eat your food
until you return to the ground. . . ."

Experience tells us that there's a right way and a wrong way to do everything, and consequences follow our actions. We cannot manage sin on our own, or in our own strength; but lessons taught by the Holy Spirit can teach us how to trust and obey. The Bible excels at sharing God's precepts by example, so let's examine what went wrong with the fall of Man in the Garden of Eden, and what went right with the bitter-sweet victory of Jesus Christ in the Garden of Gethsemane.

The Garden of Eden, which in Hebrew means *place of pleasure,* was a very special place on Earth. It was perfect. It was abundant. Yet in the midst of all its splendor and beauty . . . there was temptation.

After the serpent spoke to Eve, she turned her attention to the tree of the knowledge of Good and Evil. Genesis 3:6 shows us that the forbidden fruit appealed to Eve in three specific ways:

When the woman saw that the fruit of the tree was [1] **good for food,** [2] **pleasing to the eye** and [3] **desirable for gaining wisdom**, she took some and ate it. She also gave some to her husband, who was with her, and he ate it.

As revealed in Genesis 2:9, like God, Eve saw that the fruit was good for food and pleasing to the eye. But the third element — desirable for gaining wisdom — became the ultimate temptation. All the trees and plants on Earth were good and pleasing, but this one offered a God-like quality Adam and Eve did not possess.

With the seed of doubt firmly planted, Eve made up her mind that the fruit of that tree could fulfill three legitimate human appetites: food, beauty, and wisdom. In the blink of an eye, pride, covetousness, and disobedience replaced humble submission and trust.

Incidentally, Ezekiel tells us Satan committed these exact sins against God: *"In the pride of your heart you say, "I am a god..."* (28:2), with special mention of his fall depicted in verses 12-17:

> *You were the seal of perfection, full of wisdom and perfect in beauty.*
>
> - *You were in Eden, the garden of God; every precious stone adorned you: carnelian, chrysolite and emerald, topaz, onyx and jasper, lapis lazuli, turquoise and beryl.*
> - *Your settings and mountings were made of gold; on the day you were created they were prepared.*
> - *You were anointed as a guardian cherub, for so I ordained you.*
> - *You were on the holy mount of God; you walked among the fiery stones.*
> - *You were blameless in your ways from the day you were created till wickedness was found in you.*
> - *Through your widespread trade you were filled with violence, and you sinned.*
> - *So I drove you in disgrace from the mount of God, and I expelled you, guardian cherub, from among the fiery stones.*
> - *Your heart became proud on account of your beauty, and you corrupted your wisdom because of your splendor.*

Before the formation of the universe, Satan was an angel, a guardian cherub, whom God created. Given free will to choose whether or not he would obey God, he chose to disobey and was expelled from God's presence, along with the angels that followed him. Satan then conspired to have Adam and Eve (who were made in God's image and who ruled over the earth) expelled as well, and he used food, appetites, desires, and pride as the means to tempt mankind into committing sin.

But why would Satan want Adam and Eve to be separated from God's presence? Pride, envy, and vindictiveness. Isaiah 14:13-14 tells us: *Thou hast said in thy heart (spirit), I will ascend into heaven, I will exalt my throne above the stars of God. . . . I will ascend above the heights of the clouds; I will be like the most High (God)."* Because of his pride, Satan wanted to destroy the relationship between God and His creation. He wanted to separate God from those He loves, to sentence mankind to death. He wants us to join him.

Misery loves company. Scripture reveals the ultimate fates of Satan and his fallen angels:

> *God did not spare angels when they sinned, but sent them to hell, putting them in chains of darkness to be held for judgment. . . .*
>
> 2 Peter 2:4

> *The angels who did not keep their positions of authority but abandoned their proper dwelling — these he has kept in darkness, bound with everlasting chains for judgment on the great Day.*
>
> Jude 1:6

What we learn from these passages is this: The devil and his angels are destined for judgment and destruction; no pardon will ever be offered. But for those made in God's image, the free gifts of grace, mercy, and forgiveness await.

Those who acknowledge Jesus Christ as their Savior are given new life. If you truly believe Christ paid the ultimate price for your sin with His precious blood, our loving God offers you forgiveness, eternal life, and His Holy Spirit as your counselor and source of wisdom and knowledge. In fact, the Spirit teaches believers how to keep all fleshly appetites under control and in balance!

We see an illustration of the Holy Spirit's powerful teaching in Jesus, as He modeled the lesson of controlling fleshly appetites throughout His ministry. When it came to the greatest temptation of all, sacrificing one's life to save others, Jesus demonstrated this precept perfectly in the Garden of Gethsemane.

Gethsemane, which in Hebrew means "oil press" or "place of crushing," was east of Jerusalem, near the foot of the Mount of Olives. Jesus' anguish and betrayal took place in this garden the night before His crucifixion.

Jesus went with his disciples to a place called Gethsemane. And he said to them, "Sit here while I go over there to pray." He took Peter and the two sons of Zebedee along with him, and he began to be sorrowful and troubled. Then he said to them, "My soul is overwhelmed with sorrow to the point of death. Stay here and keep watch with me."

Going a little further, he fell with his face to the ground and prayed, "My father, if it is possible, may this cup be taken from me. Yet not as I will, but as you will."

Matthew 26:36-39

Three of the four Gospels record Jesus' vehement prayers, cries, and pleas to God to spare Him from the cup of having to experience separation from His Eternal Father by carrying *our* sins to the cross.[4] As Son of God and the Son of Man, Jesus' temptations and desires were the same as ours, yet His focus was on obedience, to do His Father's will, not His own.

Although he was a son, he learned obedience from what he suffered and, once made perfect, he became the source of eternal salvation for all who obey him. . . .

Hebrews 5:8-10

So what was God's will for mankind in the beginning? To enjoy His creation. In Nancy Guthrie's renowned book, *Jesus, Keep Me Near the Cross*, we read,

. . . the place intended for man's total enjoyment and pleasure (Garden of Eden) brought about the need for Our Lord's crushing and pain (Garden of Gethsemane). But thank God for his willingness to be "bruised for our iniquities" for "by His stripes we are healed."

In Eden, Adam sinned. In Gethsemane, the Savior overcame sin.

In Eden, Adam fell. In Gethsemane, Jesus conquered.

In Eden, Adam hid himself. In Gethsemane, our Lord boldly presented himself.

In Eden, the sword was drawn. In Gethsemane, it was sheathed.[5]

Jesus died so that you could enjoy life, in both Heaven and here on earth: *"I have come that they may have life, and have it to the full"* (John 10:10).

In the Garden of Gethsemane, Jesus made up His mind to do His Father's will — no matter what. The result: A death sentence and resurrection that would ultimately offer rebirth, glory and eternal life to those who believed in Him.

In the Garden of Eden, Adam and Eve made up their minds to disregard God's will and follow Satan's lead.

Today, you and I carry on the consequences of their actions — and our own — into many areas of our lives, including our eating.

But what Adam and Eve lost, Jesus restored, and we are called to pluck precious lessons from both gardens. First, to learn lessons from Adam and Eve's *wrong* example, then follow Jesus' *right* example.

Wrong thinking triggers wrong eating, so the first step is to *be transformed by the renewing of your mind. Then you will be able to test and approve what God's will is — his good, pleasing and perfect will"* (Romans 12:2).

By submitting to His good, pleasing, and perfect will, you can experience a genesis of your own through the power and mind of Christ Jesus and His Holy Spirit who guides you.

God formed us. Sin deformed us. Christ transforms us.

In this study, we'll use an original Recipe for a Healthy and Holy Hunger that will strengthen and encourage you on your journey to transformation. The six key ingredients are:

Prayer & Devotion • Attitude • Hospitality • Discipline • Perseverance • Accountability

Prayer & Devotion

At Jesus' birth, his mother, Mary, placed Him in a manger, which is a feeding trough for animals. Unbeknownst to Mary, Jesus came to feed us. Each day, we need to implement this truth in our lives. Daily spending time devoted in prayer with the Lord — feeding our spirits with His Word — is the first step to growing a relationship with Him and demonstrating a desire for change.

When your words came, I ate them; they were my joy and my heart's delight, for I bear your name, O Lord God Almighty.

Jeremiah 15:16

I have not departed from the commands of his lips; I have treasured the words of His mouth more than my daily bread.

Job 23:12

I am the LORD your God. . . . Open wide your mouth and I will fill it.

Psalm 81:10

They received the message with great eagerness and examined the Scriptures every day to see if what Paul said was true.

Acts 17:11

Attitude

Eating and drinking with a worshipful attitude directly affects the body, soul and spirit:

May the God who gives endurance and encouragement give you the same attitude of mind toward each other that Christ Jesus had. . . .

Romans 15:5

The word of God is alive and active. Sharper than any double-edged sword, it penetrates even to dividing soul and spirit, joints and marrow; it judges the thoughts and attitudes of the heart.

Hebrews 4:12

Hospitality

By being wise stewards of the resources God has provided, we allow our homes and tables to become places of blessing to all who enter.

Share with God's people who are in need. Practice hospitality.

Romans 12:13

They broke bread in their homes and ate together with glad and sincere hearts. . . .

Acts 2:46

Discipline

For a Christian, discipline is an inseparable aspect of who we are. In fact, the word *Christian* is simply another name for a disciple of Christ (Acts 11:26), and the word *disciple* is a branch form of the root word *discipline*. So discipline and being a disciple (or Christian) go hand in hand!

Blessed is the one whom God corrects; so do not despise the discipline of the Almighty.

Job 5:17

I discipline my body and make it my slave, so that, after I have preached to others, I myself will not be disqualified.

1 Corinthians 9:27 NASB

Perseverance

You are the beloved child of God, adopted by the Father, betrothed to the Son and empowered by the Holy Spirit. This truth defines who you are and enables you to persevere in your struggles.

You need to persevere so that when you have done the will of God, you will receive what He has promised.

Hebrews 10:36

The seed on good soil stands for those with a noble and good heart, who hear the word, retain it, and by persevering produce a good crop.

Luke 8:15

And last, but never least . . .

Accountability

We cannot do this on our own. A mature, trusted, and godly accountability partner is essential for growth in all the right areas. Solomon summed it up perfectly:

Two are better than one, because they have a good return for their work; if one falls down, his friend can help him up. But pity the man who falls and has no one to help him up! . . . A cord of three strands is not quickly broken.

Ecclesiastes 4:9-12

Encourage one another daily, as long as it is called "Today," so that none of you may be hardened by sin's deceitfulness.

Hebrews 3:13

Keep this one thing in mind throughout this study:

Being a Christian is not a self-improvement program. It is a transformation and a sanctification of your daily life through His Spirit over a lifetime.

As the saying goes, "If God brings you to it, He will bring you through it!"

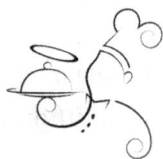

Mise en Place

Lose Sin – Gain Christ!

Prayer/Devotion • *Attitude* • *Hospitality* • *Discipline* • *Perseverance* • *Accountability*

One of the most difficult activities I had to train myself to embrace while cooking is the discipline of *mise en place*. Pronounced "MEEZ-ahn-plahs," the French term simply means to "put in place." Before you start cooking, you get everything ready: Ingredients are measured out, washed, chopped, and placed in individual bowls. Equipment and utensils, such as spatulas and blenders, pots and pans, are prepared for use, and ovens are preheated. Mise en place can make all the difference between an enjoyable, leisurely cooking experience and hectic chaos caused because the ingredients are being gathered and prepared at the same time as the recipe is being cooked.

The same principle applies with our Recipe for Healthy and Holy Hunger. Each lesson of this study supplies you with the key seven ingredients listed above to help you "put in place" what you need in order to Lose Sin and Gain Christ.

For this first lesson's mise en place, look up the scriptural references below and answer the questions in the spaces provided. Then, for the next seven days munch on and memorize (by heart) each passage. As you do this, you'll not only grow in the knowledge of God, you'll nourish your mind, body, soul, and spirit.

1) **Genesis 1:30:** In the perfect Garden of Eden, what was the first type of food God gave to man?

   _____

2) **Genesis 9:3-4:** After the flood, what did God give as food to Noah, his family and mankind?

   _____

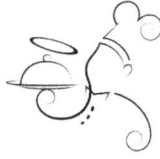

3) **Mark 7:18-19:** Can we really eat *anything* we want?

_____

4) **Luke 10:8:** What should we do with food that is put before us when we are a guest at someone's home?

_____

5) **Luke 12:22-23:** We often stress over food — either for the lack of it or because we overindulge. What did Jesus say to his disciples on this topic?

_____

_____

6) **Romans 14:20-21:** Some people try to "derail" others. What does the Apostle Paul say about eating and tempting others?

_____

_____

7) **1 Corinthians 10:31:** What does Jesus want us to do above all when making food choices?

_____

Forbidden Apple, Walnut and Blue Cheese Salad with a Raspberry Vinaigrette

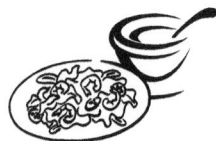

Keep my commands and you will live;
guard my teachings as the apple of your eye.

Proverb 7:2

I discovered this recipe in a cooking class and loved the heavenly combination of mixed greens with Red Delicious apples, crunchy toasted walnuts, pungent blue cheese and homemade raspberry vinaigrette. (Resist the temptation to purchase commercial dressings).

The good news: It is not a sin to eat it.

Ingredients

For all recipes contained in this study, God's Kitchen Ministries encourages the use of Certified Organic/Raw foods to maximize nutrition and gain the most health benefits.

- 1 head Romaine lettuce, a bundle of watercress, and a small bundle of chicory, washed, dried and torn into bite-size pieces
- 6 ounces blue cheese, crumbled
- 2 firm Red Delicious apples, diced
- 1 cup toasted walnuts
- ½ cup (or to taste) raspberry vinaigrette*

Instructions

Combine the Romaine, watercress and chicory with the blue cheese, apples, and walnuts in a large bowl. Toss with the raspberry vinaigrette just before serving.

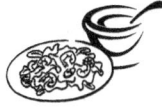

*Raspberry Vinaigrette

Ingredients

- 1 tablespoon Dijon mustard
- ¼ cup raspberry vinegar
- 1 shallot, finely chopped
- ½ cup olive oil
- ¼ cup salad oil
- salt and pepper to taste

Instructions

Combine the mustard, vinegar and shallots in a bowl and gradually whisk in the oils. Reserve the dressing until ready to use as directed.

Yield: 6 servings (Serving size: about ¾ cup)

For recipe photo and nutritional information, visit www.Gods-Kitchen.org.

Notes

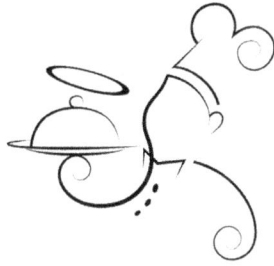

WHAT'S YOUR BEEF?

Three Attitudes: Cain, Abel, and Noah

In our first lesson, we discovered the origins of food struggles (pride, envy, and disobedience) and examined the wrong way and right way (submission, trust, and obedience) to please God. The first key ingredient in our Recipe for a Healthy and Holy Hunger — *Prayer and Devotion* —enables us to rely on our internal counselor, the Holy Spirit, and God's Word to open our hearts and allow these scriptural food revelations to become ingrained in our being.

The second ingredient in the recipe is *Attitude.* Through the lives of Cain, Abel, and Noah, we'll expand our study to observe right and wrong food-related attitudes.

In 1974, the Burger King restaurant chain launched a new motto: Have It Your Way. Advertisements for the hamburger giant included a memorable jingle with the words "Hold the pickle, hold the lettuce . . . *Have it your way . . . .*" encouraging diners to dictate the way they wanted their burgers.

Because we each have our personal preferences, choices and options can be a blessing. But what happens when this element is applied where it shouldn't be, as with Adam and Eve's choices?

When God confronted them as to what they had done, Adam got an attitude: *"The woman you put here with me — she gave me some fruit from the tree, and I ate it."*[6] Then

Eve pointed to the snake saying, *"The serpent deceived me, and I ate."*[7]

Do you recall what food options were available to them in the beginning? A delectable, diverse, incredibly satisfying, and endless all-you-can-eat worldwide buffet, compliments of the Master Chef.

Bad choices and attitudes continue to spill into many areas of our own lives today. So, before we proceed, I encourage you to begin with a word of prayer and ask the Lord to help put your 'tude about food to the side as we come before His throne of grace.

> Father God, I open all the secret places of my heart to you and say, "Come in." Jesus, I want you to be the Lord of my life — I hold nothing back. I want Your ways to be my ways. I ask Your Holy Spirit to bring me deeper into fellowship with You during this study, and to help me "let go and let God!" I echo the words of the Psalmist, *"Your ways, God, are holy. What god is as great as our God?"* (77:13). Oh Lord, I praise and thank you for the daily bread you graciously provide each and every day. By the power of Christ Jesus I pray, Amen.

Do It God's Way

Let's read from Genesis, Chapter 4:1-8

> *Adam made love to his wife Eve, and she became pregnant and gave birth to Cain. She said, "With the help of the LORD I have brought forth a man." Later she gave birth to his brother Abel.*
>
> *Now Abel kept flocks, and Cain worked the soil. In the course of time Cain brought some of the fruits of the soil as an offering to the LORD. And Abel also brought an offering — fat portions from some of the firstborn of his flock. The LORD looked with favor on Abel and his offering, but on Cain and his offering he did not look with favor. So Cain was very angry, and his face was downcast.*
>
> *Then the LORD said to Cain, "Why are you angry? Why is your face downcast? If you do what is right, will you not be accepted? But if you do not do what is right, sin is crouching at your door; it desires to have you, but you must rule over it."*
>
> *Now Cain said to his brother Abel, "Let's go out to the field." While they were in the field, Cain attacked his brother Abel and killed him.*

Both Cain and Abel had brought God the fruits of their vocations: Abel was a shepherd; Cain was a farmer. The issue concerning the individual offerings relates not only to *what* they brought to God, but also to the *attitude* with which they approached God.

Why would God accept one offering, but not the other? Dr. David Crabtree, co-author of *The Language of God: A Commonsense Approach to Understanding and Applying the Bible*, offers this commentary:

> Presumably Cain and Abel were both acutely aware of the degree to which their well being was dependent on the gracious provision by God. They were both moved to express their gratitude by "returning" to him some of what he had provided. It makes sense then that each presented an offering from that which they had produced with the gracious help of God. At this point, however, the text indicates a difference between the offerings of Cain and those of Abel — they selected that portion which they would offer to God by different criteria. Cain just presented some of what he produced to God; it was, at best, a random sampling. Abel was much more deliberate. He selected some of his firstlings and some of the "fat" portions. I believe "fat portions" is being used figuratively here. It means the best or choice portion (this same Hebrew word *chelev* is used in this sense in Numbers 18:12).
>
> In other words, rather than taking a random sampling of what he produced, Abel goes through his flock and selects the very best to present as an offering to God. This difference in method of selection betrays a difference in **attitudes** towards God." This is why the author of Hebrews (Chapter 11, verse 4) can say, "By faith Abel offered to God a better sacrifice than Cain, through which he obtained the testimony that he was righteous, God testifying about his gifts, and through faith, though he is dead he still speaks."[8]

Some commentaries say the reason God rejected Cain's offering and accepted Abel's had to do with blood sacrifice, as God later ordained in the Old Testament law. On this subject, Crabtree continues . . .

> Some have argued that the reason Cain's offering was rejected and Abel's was accepted is because Abel's offering involved the shedding of blood and this is what is necessary for forgiveness of sins. I think this is not the meaning of the text. There is no indication from the text that the

two men had been commanded by God to make offerings nor that God had given them instructions as to how to do it. It makes the most sense to assume that Cain and Abel are just trying to find an appropriate way to express thanks to God.

When God speaks to Cain, he says, "If you do well, will not your countenance be lifted up?" This seems to focus on Cain's inner disposition rather than whether or not he sacrificed an animal. If the latter had been the concern, the author would have written, "If you do the offering right. . . ." Furthermore, the word that is used to describe what they are presenting to God is "offering" rather than "sacrifice." An offering does not necessarily imply the shedding of blood; a sacrifice does. So the author is doing nothing to steer us to think in terms of a blood sacrifice being given. In the absence of such clues there is no reason to think that this is what the author intended to communicate. Therefore the meaning of the text intended by the author of Genesis does not include the idea that Abel correctly followed the rules and Cain did not.[9]

It all comes down to attitude. Does food matter more to you than God does? It certainly did to Cain. In the book *Love to Eat. Hate to Eat: Breaking the Bondage of Destructive Eating Habits*, author Elyse Fitzpatrick writes:

Let's think for a moment about the First Commandment: "Thou shalt have no other gods before me" (Exodus 20:3 KJV). Does the way that we think of food or respond to opportunities to eat function as a god for us? Remember, an idol is something that replaces God in our affections and worship. As a result, food, in a sense, has become our god: satisfying us, reassuring us, pleasing us.[10]

With that in mind, it's easy to see how our attitude toward food can easily fall into idolatry, as well as gluttony — the habitual greed of excess eating (which we will examine in another lesson).

Our primary goal should be to have an attitude of worship.

The term *worship* as derived from the old English word *wurthscipe (condition of being worthy)*, means "to acknowledge the worth of." Worship is an attitude of the heart, the response to God's worthiness, greatness, and goodness. Therefore, as Christians, when we worship God we acknowledge His worthiness.

Worship can happen every day, every hour, every minute, every time we put Him first, and every time we give Him all the glory. Psalm 9:1-2 states, *"I will give thanks to you, LORD, with all my heart; I will tell of all your wonderful deeds. I will be glad and rejoice in you; I will sing the praises of your name, O Most High."*

Now let's turn our attention to the mindset and Godly approach of the famous biblical shipbuilder, Noah. As we'll see, Noah worshipped God and was faithful to Him. And what was the result?

Let's read from Genesis, Chapters 6-8.

Chapter 6

Noah and the Flood

This is the account of Noah and his family.

Noah was a righteous man, blameless among the people of his time, and he walked faithfully with God. Noah had three sons: Shem, Ham and Japheth.

Now the earth was corrupt in God's sight and was full of violence. God saw how corrupt the earth had become, for all the people on earth had corrupted their ways. So God said to Noah, "I am going to put an end to all people, for the earth is filled with violence because of them. I am surely going to destroy both them and the earth. So make yourself an ark of cypress wood; make rooms in it and coat it with pitch inside and out. . . . I am going to bring floodwaters on the earth to destroy all life under the heavens, every creature that has the breath of life in it. Everything on earth will perish. But I will establish my covenant with you, and you will enter the ark — you and your sons and your wife and your sons' wives with you. . . . Every kind of creature that moves along the ground will come to you to be kept alive. You are to take every kind of food that is to be eaten and store it away as food for you and for them."

Noah did everything just as God commanded him.

Chapter 7

The LORD then said to Noah, "Go into the ark, you and your whole family, because I have found you righteous in this generation. . . .

And Noah did all that the LORD commanded him. . . .

In the six hundredth year of Noah's life, on the seventeenth day of the second month — on that day all the springs of the great deep burst forth, and the floodgates of the heavens were opened. And rain fell on the earth forty days and forty nights.

On that very day Noah and his sons, Shem, Ham and Japheth, together with his wife and the wives of his three sons, entered the ark. They had with them every wild animal according to its kind, all livestock according to their kinds, every creature that moves along the ground according to its kind and every bird according to its kind, everything with wings . . . Then the LORD shut him in.

For forty days the flood kept coming on the earth, and as the waters increased they lifted the ark high above the earth. . . . The waters rose and covered the mountains to a depth of more than fifteen cubits. . . . Every living thing on the face of the earth was wiped out; people and animals and the creatures that move along the ground and the birds were wiped from the earth. Only Noah was left, and those with him in the ark.

The waters flooded the earth for a hundred and fifty days.

Chapter 8

But God remembered Noah and all the wild animals and the livestock that were with him in the ark, and he sent a wind over the earth, and the waters receded. . . . At the end of the hundred and fifty days the water had gone down, and on the seventeenth day of the seventh month the ark came to rest on the mountains of Ararat. The waters continued to recede until the tenth month, and on the first day of the tenth month the tops of the mountains became visible.

After forty days Noah opened a window he had made in the ark and sent out a raven, and it kept flying back and forth until the water had dried up from the earth. Then he sent out a dove to see if the water had receded from the surface of the ground. But the dove could find nowhere to perch because there was water over all the surface of the earth; so it returned to Noah in the ark. . . . He waited seven more days and again sent out the dove from the ark. When the dove returned to him in the evening, there in its beak was a freshly plucked olive leaf! Then Noah knew that the water had receded from the earth. He waited seven more days and sent the dove out again, but this time it did not return to him.

By the first day of the first month of Noah's six hundred and first year, the water had dried up from the earth. Noah then removed the covering from the ark and saw that the surface of the ground was dry. By the twenty-seventh day of the second month the earth was completely dry.

Then God said to Noah, "Come out of the ark, you and your wife and your sons and their wives. Bring out every kind of living creature that is with you — the birds, the animals, and all the creatures that move along the ground — so they can multiply on the earth and be fruitful and increase in number on it."

So Noah came out, together with his sons and his wife and his sons' wives. All the animals and all the creatures that move along the ground and all the birds —everything that moves on land — came out of the ark, one kind after another.

Then Noah built an altar to the Lord and, taking some of all the clean animals and clean birds, he sacrificed burnt offerings on it. The Lord smelled the pleasing aroma and said in his heart: "Never again will I curse the ground because of humans, even though every inclination of the human heart is evil from childhood. And never again will I destroy all living creatures, as I have done.

"As long as the earth endures, seedtime and harvest, cold and heat, summer and winter, day and night will never cease."

Second Peter 2:5 refers to Noah as a *"preacher of righteousness."* Faithful to God's will, while he was building the ark, Noah preached for approximately one hundred and twenty years to a world that had fallen so deeply into sin that *the LORD was grieved that he had made man on the earth, and his heart was filled with pain.*[11] Unsuccessful in converting those whose *every inclination . . . was only evil all the time,*[12] Noah entered the ark with his wife, his three sons and their wives (total of eight), and all were saved from the Flood.

God blessed Noah by calling him an *heir of righteousness.*[13] From Noah's life, we learn that an attitude of *faithfulness* brings great reward.

Another notable event here should be of interest to us. It relates to the new covenant between God and Noah, and a change in dietary restrictions.

Let's read from Genesis, Chapter 9, verses 1-7

Then God blessed Noah and his sons, saying to them, "Be fruitful and increase in number and fill the earth. The fear and dread of you will fall on all the beasts of the earth, and on all the birds in the sky, on every creature that moves along the ground, and on all the fish in the sea; they are given into your hands. Everything that lives and moves about will be food for you. Just as I gave you the green plants, I now give you everything.

"But you must not eat meat that has its lifeblood still in it. And for your lifeblood I will surely demand an accounting. I will demand an accounting from every animal. And from each human being, too, I will demand an accounting for the life of another human being.

"Whoever sheds human blood, by humans shall their blood be shed; for in the image of God has God made mankind. As for you, be fruitful and increase in number; multiply on the earth and increase upon it."

God told Noah, as He had Adam and Eve, to be fruitful and multiply; but something changed. In Genesis 1:29, we saw that God told Adam and Eve, "*I give you every seed-bearing plant on the face of the whole earth and every tree that has fruit with seed in it. They will be yours for food.*" But in Genesis 9:3 we see God tell Noah, "*Everything that lives and moves will be food for you. Just as I gave you the green plants, I now give you everything.*"

Until this point, the Bible makes no mention of eating meat. This is the first time we see "everything that lives and moves" mentioned as food. This text is subject to great debate and controversy, so we will briefly discuss two major points that relate to both food and attitude:

First: As the earth was flooded, the food supply of plants and trees would have been affected. John Woodmorappe, author of *Noah's Ark: A Feasibility Study*, writes:

The Flood was an ecological catastrophe. Creationists credit it with eroding and redepositing sediments miles thick, raising mountains, carving immense canyons, and even repositioning continents. This alone would doom many plants to extinction, even if they or their seeds survived the Flood, for some of the following reasons:

40

- Most of the world's seeds would have been buried under many feet — even miles — of sediment. This would keep them from sprouting.

- Many plants require particular soil conditions to grow. The Flood would have eroded away all the topsoil which provides the optimum conditions for most plants.

- Some seeds will germinate only after being exposed to fire. After the Flood, there was nothing to burn.

- Most flowering plants are pollinated by insects, but the only insects around after the Flood would have been those Noah carried aboard the ark. The surviving seeds would have had to find the proper conditions of soil type and burial depth in a small area around where the ark landed.

- Plants live not as individuals, but as communities. If you cut down the redwoods, you kill not only the redwoods but also dozens of other plants that depend on the community structure. After the Flood, there would have been no ecological communities, only bare land. Any plant that depends on a mature community (for shade, shelter, humidity, or support, for example) could not survive until such a community matures, which usually takes years to decades.[14]

Second: In Genesis 9:4 God made a stipulation: "*You must not eat meat that has its lifeblood still in it.*"

Historically, pagans drank blood in connection with their worship rituals and ceremonies. They believed drinking the blood of an animal, or even of their enemies, would give them the strength of whatever they killed and would keep them young and strong.

Whatever, or whoever, we worship in this life will bind us . . . will yoke us. Romans 6:16 clearly states this: *Don't you know that when you offer yourselves to someone as obedient slaves, you are slaves of the one you obey — whether you are slaves to sin, which leads to death, or to obedience, which leads to righteousness?*

And in Luke 16:13 we learn that *no servant can serve two masters: for either he will hate the one, and love the other; or else he will hold to the one, and despise the other . . . .*

Jesus said in Matthew 11:29-30, *"Take my yoke upon you and learn from me, for I am gentle and humble in heart, and you will find rest for your souls. For my yoke is easy and my burden is light."*

What does it mean to take the yoke of Jesus upon us? It means to be bound to or joined with Christ, to walk with Christ in a manner that pleases Him, never rushing ahead (to do anything without His leading) or lagging behind when He calls to follow. Through Christ, the yoke (bond) of slavery is broken and the blessed yoke to our Creator is restored. Sadly, few are willing to accept it. An ox is forced by its owner to take the yoke upon its neck. But Jesus invites us, without compulsion.

Why would anyone reject this kind of invitation? Because they would rather take the heavy yoke of their self-will (independence) — with its frustrations, defeats, and regrets — than the light yoke of Jesus (obedience) that brings true liberty and deep rest.

Worship is the new beginning we all need to put an end to our struggles with sin. When we worship God, we admit our weakness and inadequacies and rely on His strength and grace to teach us how to live . . . and how to eat. However, it is important to understand that we do not worship God in weakness and inadequacy, for we . . . *approach God's throne of grace with confidence, so that we may receive mercy and find grace to help us in our time of need* (Hebrews 4:16).

Remember to put on an attitude of worship, draw near to God with all your heart, and praise Him with the fruit of your lips!

Notes

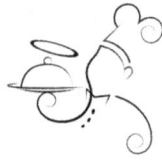

Mise en Place

Lose Sin – Gain Christ!

*Prayer/Devotion • **Attitude** • Hospitality • Discipline • Perseverance • Accountability*

Understanding the Lord's purpose and approach to food is vital to recognizing the importance of our own attitude toward food. Once again, look up the scriptural references below and answer the questions in the spaces provided. Then, for the next seven days munch on and memorize (by heart) each passage so you can grow in the knowledge of God and nourish your mind, body, soul and spirit.

1) **Matthew 4:4:** What is more important than food?

_____

_____

2) **Matthew 6:25:** What are you not to worry about?

_____

_____

3) **In light of the above,** what do you think Jesus really wants your attitude and approach to food to be?

_____

_____

4) **1 Corinthians 6:13:** What is food for and what will be the end result?

_____

_____

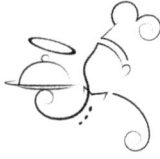

5) **1 Corinthians 8:8:** What can food not do?

_____

_____

6) **1 Timothy 4:1-4:** Our culture is obsessed with diet crazes that limit our food selections. Does God put limits on what kinds of food we can eat? What should we do throughout the day with what we are given?

_____

_____

7) **Ezra 6:22:** What does this scripture tell you about God's spirit? Is anything impossible for the Lord?

_____

_____

Noah's Tender Cow Carne on a Raft

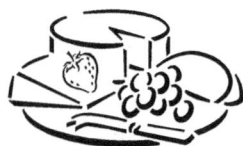

Everything that lives and moves will be food for you.
Just as I gave you the green plants, I now give you everything.

Genesis 9:3

The original name of this recipe is Grilled Beef Tenderloin Crostini with Mustard-Horseradish Sauce, but use whatever name floats your boat! It's a great, healthy appetizer that is fun to make, looks impressive when served, and ensures "meat eaters" will be well satisfied.

Ingredients

For all recipes contained in this study, God's Kitchen Ministries encourages the use of Certified Organic/Raw foods to maximize nutrition and gain the most health benefits.

- ⅔ cup sour cream
- ¼ cup Dijon mustard
- 1 tablespoon horseradish
- 2 tablespoons fresh tarragon, finely chopped
- 1½ pounds cooked beef tenderloin (grilled or roasted)
- ½ teaspoon freshly ground black pepper
- 2 tablespoons fresh lemon juice
- 1 bunch of arugula
- 1 (8 ounce) French baguette, cut diagonally into 16 slices
- 2 tablespoons capers
- ½ cup (2 ounces) fresh Parmesan cheese, shaved

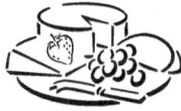

Instructions

Combine the sour cream with the mustard, horseradish, and chopped tarragon, stirring well with a whisk. Cover and chill.

Slice the beef tenderloin thinly, then lightly sprinkle with black pepper and lemon juice.

Arrange the arugula over the slices of bread, then top with one beef slice and about one tablespoon of the mustard cream.

Sprinkle the capers and Parmesan cheese evenly over the top.

Yield: 16 servings (Serving size: 1 sandwich)

For recipe photo and nutritional information, visit www.Gods-Kitchen.org.

Notes

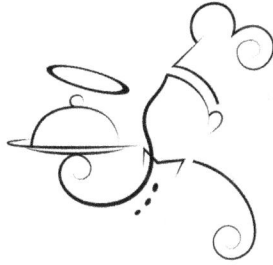

ENTERTAINING ANGELS —
PURSUING HOSPITALITY

As we slice and dice our way into the third lesson, two of the ingredients for our Recipe for a Healthy and Holy Hunger have already been weighed and measured: *Prayer and Devotion*, and *Attitude*. We now open the proverbial kitchen cupboard to reveal our next biblical ingredient: the spiritual discipline of *Hospitality*.

When you think of modern-day hospitality, what comes to mind? Entertaining family or friends? Martha Stewart, perhaps? When we reduce hospitality to this degree, we forfeit biblical understanding. In Scripture, hospitality is not merely the practice of entertaining guests; it is a way of life, a Christ-centered ethic, and a preview of the coming of God's Kingdom.

The purpose of this lesson is to see the role of food and hospitality in a new light. Combined, these crucial elements expand our reach with others and empower us in God's service.

First, let's pause to open with a word of prayer to God Our Heavenly Father, *Abba*.[15]

> Lord, as I examine this study, may Your love shine through my life as I learn how to practice the spiritual discipline of hospitality. Teach me how to create opportunities to offer what I have to others. I want to share what You have provided. I thank you for all that I have and I am grateful that Your Spirit is

always with me. Bless me, Lord, with a generous heart to use my gifts, my provisions, and my home for Your good purposes. In Jesus' Name, Amen.

Let's read Genesis, Chapter 18:1-8

Note: If you are not familiar with the history of Abram/Abraham, the Great Patriarch of the People of Israel, I encourage you to also read Genesis Chapters 12-18 in your Bible.

The Three Visitors

The LORD appeared to Abraham near the great trees of Mamre while he was sitting at the entrance to his tent in the heat of the day. Abraham looked up and saw three men standing nearby. When he saw them, he hurried from the entrance of his tent to meet them and bowed low to the ground.

He said, "If I have found favor in your eyes, my lord, do not pass your servant by. Let a little water be brought, and then you may all wash your feet and rest under this tree. Let me get you something to eat, so you can be refreshed and then go on your way — now that you have come to your servant."

"Very well," they answered, "do as you say."

So Abraham hurried into the tent to Sarah. "Quick," he said, "get three seahs of the finest flour and knead it and bake some bread."

Then he ran to the herd and selected a choice, tender calf and gave it to a servant, who hurried to prepare it. He then brought some curds and milk and the calf that had been prepared, and set these before them. While they ate, he stood near them under a tree.

Abraham and the "Tree" Visitors

If we could go back in time to Chapter 18, this is what we might see:

It is mid-day. Abraham is sitting near the entrance to his tent, peering out through the shimmering heat waves of the desert sun when, suddenly, he sees three men at the great trees of Mamre. They have not arrived by camel (remember, they are in the desert), they have just appeared out of nowhere and are standing in the nearby shade.

Their sudden appearance during the hottest time of the day is startling. Immediately,

Abraham shifts into high gear and becomes a model of true hospitality. He runs to them as if they are long-lost relatives, bows down in reverence, and greets them like royalty.

Why? Who are these unexpected visitors? The Lord Almighty and two angels! Abraham extends an invitation to dine, saying that it would be his privilege to serve them. The menu is modest and the accommodation humble: just a little water to wash the dust off their sandaled feet, and a tree serving as a canopy for shade and rest. Abraham will fetch a morsel of bread. It will only take a few minutes, and then they can go on their way.

How can they refuse such simple kindness?

Their answer is brief, a mere four words in Hebrew: *"Do as you say."*

With permission thus granted, Abraham is on a mission. He hurries back to his tent.

In biblical times, hospitality was a sacred duty, an obligation to receive, feed, lodge, and protect *any* traveler who might knock at your door. It played an important role in tribal and domestic life. Life in the desert made this type of hospitality necessary for survival, and among the nomads it became a highly esteemed virtue. Through hospitality, the stranger or weary traveler found rest, food, shelter, and protection. He was treated as an honored guest, and the men who ate together became bound to each other by the strongest ties of friendship. This friendship was passed down to their children . . . and their children's children.

Remarkably, Bedouins still maintain this same practice in the desert today.

The Greek word for hospitality is *philoxenia*. This word is comprised of *xenos*, "stranger," and *phileo*, "to love or show affection." So the word literally means "to love strangers." According to Definitions.net,[16] the definition of hospitality is "the act or practice of one who is hospitable; receptive, and entertainment of strangers or guests without reward, or with kind and generous liberality."

In our modern culture hospitality has, regretfully, taken on a more closed-door approach. Although the act of cooking dinners for family and church friends and family is a gracious thing to do, it is not an example of biblical hospitality.

Have you ever extended the hand of hospitality to a total stranger or to someone who was desperately in need? It is an awesome, gratifying experience.

Several years ago, I was a single parent and the leader of our church's single adult's ministry. As the Thanksgiving holiday was fast approaching, I decided to invite a few single friends over to my home to share the feast. The morning before the event, I opened my Bible and the Lord spoke directly to my heart from Scripture:

> *Then Jesus said to his host, "When you give a luncheon or dinner, do not invite your friends, your brothers or sisters, your relatives, or your rich neighbors; if you do, they may invite you back and so you will be repaid. But when you give a banquet, invite the poor, the crippled, the lame, the blind, and you will be blessed. Although they cannot repay you, you will be repaid at the resurrection of the righteous."*
>
> Luke 14:12

His wishes were loud and clear: Extend an invitation for Thanksgiving to someone in need. But who, I wondered? In truth, I was a bit nervous, but I decided I would pray for the Lord's direction and follow through when the opportunity presented itself. That very afternoon, I stepped into Starbucks for my usual, and noticed the barista who always attended to my order was handicapped. Spiritually prompted, I asked him what his plans were for Thanksgiving and I discovered he was going to be alone on the holiday. When I extended the invitation to dinner, he accepted with a huge smile. Those are what I call "God Moments." To date, it is one of my best Thanksgiving memories — all because the Lord spoke to my heart and I obeyed. That year, God taught me the true meaning of selfless, biblical hospitality.

But this gift of service is not just about (or limited to) preparing and offering *food*. Scripture shows us several examples of hospitality.

In Genesis 19, Abraham's nephew, Lot, protected his two guests — God's angels — from the townsmen who surrounded the house and made threats. Here, hospitality is associated with *protection*.

Similarly, in Joshua 2 Rahab offered protection and lodging to Israelite spies, demonstrating her loyalty to Israel's God. In 1 Samuel 25, Abigail provided hospitality to David and his men. In 1 Kings 17, the widow of Zarephath provided hospitality for Elijah when she was facing starvation, prompting God to provide for her.

Hospitality is a characteristic of those who live as God intends. Again and again, actions reveal the good or evil of a person or a community (Genesis 19, Judges 19, and 1 Samuel 25). The same is true in the New Testament. Do you know which parable uses hospitality to demonstrate loving our neighbor? Read the parable of the Good Samaritan (Luke 10:25-37).

How Can You Practice Biblical Hospitality?

Share with God's people who are in need. Practice hospitality.

Romans 12:13

Some other scriptural references include the following:

Let us not become weary in doing good, for at the proper time we will reap a harvest if we do not give up.

Galatians 6:9

We ought therefore to show hospitality to such people so that we may work together for the truth.

3 John: 8

What good is it, my brothers and sisters, if someone claims to have faith but has no deeds? Can such faith save them? Suppose a brother or a sister is without clothes and daily food. If one of you says to them, "Go in peace; keep warm and well fed," but does nothing about their physical needs, what good is it?

James 2:14-16

If anyone has material possessions and sees a brother or sister in need but has no pity on them, how can the love of God be in that person? Dear children, let us not love with words or speech but with actions and in truth.

1 John 3:17-18

Above all, love each other deeply, because love covers over a multitude of sins. Offer hospitality to one another without grumbling. Each of you should use whatever gift you have received to serve others, as faithful stewards of God's grace in its various forms.

1 Peter 4:8-10

Jesus reached out to *thousands* of strangers in need: the hungry, the sick, the rich, and the poor. He practiced hospitality when he fed the multitudes (Mark 6:30-44).

He accepted hospitality from Simon the Pharisee and a Pharisee ruler (Luke 10:38-42, Matthew 26:6-13) as well as Zacchaeus and the Emmaus host (Luke 19:5, Luke 24:29).

Are we not called to do the same?

And what does the Lord say will be our ultimate reward?

"The King will say to those on his right, 'Come, you who are blessed by my Father, inherit the kingdom prepared for you from the foundation of the world. For I was hungry and you gave me food, I was thirsty and you gave me drink, I was a stranger and you welcomed me, I was naked and you clothed me, I was sick and you visited me, I was in prison and you came to me.' Then the righteous will answer him, saying, 'Lord, when did we see you hungry and feed you, or thirsty and give you drink? And when did we see you a stranger and welcome you, or naked and clothe you? And when did we see you sick or in prison and visit you?' And the King will answer them, 'Truly, I say to you, as you did it to one of the least of these my brothers, you did it to me.'"

Matthew 25:34-46

I'll close today's lesson with a poem by American satirist, Ambrose Gwinnett Bierce:

HOSPITALITY

Why ask me, Gastrogogue, to dine,
Unless to praise your rascal wine.
Yet never ask some luckless sinner
Who needs, as I do not, a dinner?[17]

Hospitality is a wonderful gift. When we offer our food or extend hospitality to just those close to us, we lose the distinctive nature of Christ-like discipleship.

You do not need an impressive home to make others feel welcome — just an open heart. As we're told in Hebrews 13:2: *Do not forget to entertain strangers, for by so doing some people have entertained angels without knowing it.*

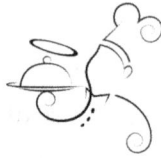

Mise en Place

Lose Sin – Gain Christ!

*Prayer/Devotion • Attitude • **Hospitality** • Discipline • Perseverance • Accountability*

Below is a "cooked up" version of author Patricia A. Ennis' HOSPITALITY acrostic word collage[18] that outlines what a person of Christian character, who desires to practice biblical hospitality, might look like.

Research each scripture reference and note it in the space provided.

A Person Of Christian Character Who Practices Biblical Hospitality Is . . .

H — Humble

Humility is the opposite of self-sufficiency and is a necessary prerequisite . . . to be of service to God. We can exercise humility by choosing to step out of our "comfort zones" and invite individuals into our home with whom we may not be totally at ease.

1 Peter 5:5

_____

_____

O — Obedient

The primary evidence that individuals are Christians is their choice to obey God's commands.

1 Samuel 15:22

_____

_____

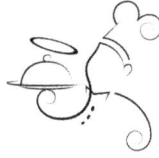

S — Sincere

"Genuine," as well as an "absence of deceit or hypocrisy," describes sincere actions; be sure to extend sincere invitations.

2 Corinthians 1:12

_____

_____

P — Prayerful

Communication with your Heavenly Father, shows your desire for His direction and your dependence on Him. Resolve to pray about everything, including all aspects of the events you plan.

1 Thessalonians 5:17

_____

_____

I — Integrity

Integrity is choosing to do what is right when given a choice between right and wrong, even when it is unpopular. Choose to adhere to God's standards, regardless of what the mainstream of society is doing.

Psalm 25:21

_____

_____

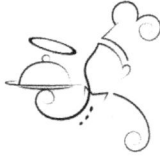

T — Trustworthy

A trustworthy home provides an ambience of trust and confidence.

Proverb 31:11

_____

_____

A — Adopted into God's Family

Adoption is making a conscious choice to legally integrate an individual into another's home and nurture them as if they were a biological child. Behave in a way that reflects your royal heritage, so that your guests will observe a bit of "heaven on earth" in your home!

Romans 8:15

_____

_____

L — Led by the Spirit

Keeping in step and allowing Him to lead you so you do not carry out the desire of your flesh.

Romans 8:14, Galatians 5:16-18

_____

_____

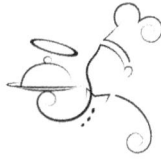

I — Instrumental in Producing Righteousness

Bringing "every thought captive to the obedience of Christ" and refusing to worry about anything. God has empowered us to control what we think and to be spiritually renewed by presenting our concerns to Him . . . even when things appear to be beyond our capabilities.

2 Corinthians 10:5, Philippians 4:6-8, Romans 6:13

T — Thankful

Being thankful is an act of the will that generates the giving of thanks to God — regardless of the circumstances.

Colossians 3:17

Y — Yielded

Possessing a willingness to yield to my heavenly Father's specific instructions to His children in relation to practicing hospitality. I demonstrate my love to Him by choosing to embrace His instructions with my whole heart — and that is when my joy is complete.

Romans 6:19, 1 John 1:4, 2 John 12

Divine Pumpkin Streusel Bread

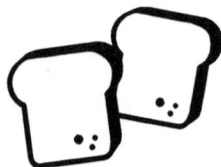

*"Let me get you something to eat,
so you can be refreshed and then go on your way. . . ."*

Genesis 18:5

In the Bible, when God's people offered hospitality they "broke bread."

Nothing on earth rivals the smell of homemade bread wafting through the house to welcome guests. You will be richly blessed if you make dozens of this "loaf-offering" to share with those in need.

Ingredients

For all recipes contained in this study, God's Kitchen Ministries encourages the use of Certified Organic/Raw foods to maximize nutrition and gain the most health benefits.

- ½ cup chopped pecans
- 1½ tablespoons unsalted butter, chilled
- 2 tablespoons sugar
- ¼ teaspoon ground cinnamon
- 2 cups all-purpose flour
- ½ cup sugar
- ½ cup raisins
- 1 teaspoon baking powder
- 1 teaspoon salt
- ½ teaspoon ground cinnamon
- ½ teaspoon ground cloves
- ½ teaspoon ground nutmeg
- 15 ounce can 100% pure pumpkin
- ½ cup plain or Greek yogurt
- ½ cup honey
- ½ cup vegetable oil
- 1 teaspoon vanilla
- 2 eggs, lightly beaten
- cooking spray

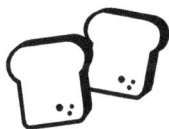

Instructions

Preheat oven to 350°.

To prepare the topping, combine the chopped pecans with the chilled butter, 2 tablespoons of sugar, and ¼ teaspoon cinnamon. The mixture should look crumbly. Set aside.

To prepare the bread, lightly spoon the flour into dry measuring cups and level with a knife. Mix with the ½ cup of sugar, raisins, baking powder, salt, and remaining spices in a large bowl, making a well in the center of the mixture.

In a separate bowl, combine the pumpkin with the yogurt, honey, vegetable oil, vanilla, and the two lightly beaten eggs.

Add this to the well in the center of the flour mixture, stirring gently until the dry ingredients have been combined and the mixture is just moist.

Spoon the batter into a 9 x 5 inch loaf pan coated with cooking spray.

Sprinkle the pecan topping over the batter.

Bake at 350° for 1 hour or until a wooden toothpick inserted into the center comes out clean.

Cool for 10 minutes before removing from the pan. Allow to cool completely on a wire rack.

Yield: 16 servings (Serving size: 1 slice)

For recipe photo and nutritional information, visit www.Gods-Kitchen.org.

Notes

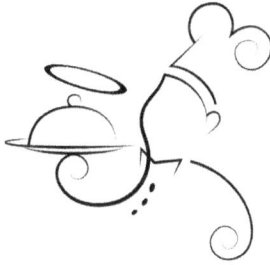

OUT-OF-CONTROL APPETITES

Mastering Sinful Appetites

The world teaches us that the way to overcome sinful and unhealthy appetites is to hold fast to a series of rules, regulations, and guidelines. Although moral absolutes provide us with solid behavioral standards, they are not the means to the ultimate end . . . as the Apostle Paul wrote to the believers living in Colossae some two thousand years ago:

> *Since you died with Christ to the elemental spiritual forces of this world, why, as though you still belonged to the world, do you submit to its rules: "Do not handle! Do not taste! Do not touch!"? These rules, which have to do with things that are all destined to perish with use, are based on merely human commands and teachings. Such regulations indeed have an appearance of wisdom, with their self-imposed worship, their false humility and their harsh treatment of the body, but they lack any value in restraining sensual indulgence.*

Colossians 2:20-23

In their purest forms, most of our appetites, desires, and urges are God-given. The trouble arises when we allow our carnal self — in this case, our stomachs — to take over His rightful place on the throne of our hearts. God wants us to depend solely on Him to seek relief and rescue from any obsession that takes control over our lives.

In this lesson, we will discuss the approach to mastering these desires through another key ingredient in our Recipe for a Healthy and Holy Hunger: *Discipline.*

Not possible, you say? Jesus would tell you: *"With man, this is impossible, but with God, all things are possible."*[19]

The first step is to admit we cannot conquer sin on our own. The next step is to ask the Lord to provide the strength we need to master it.

Heavenly Father, I have tried to do things my way and in my own strength, but I fall short time and time again. I ask for spiritual discernment as I read what Your Word says on disciplining my appetites. Make my heart hungry for the wonderful promises, provisions, and precepts revealed throughout Scripture, which you declared would not *"return to me empty, but will accomplish what I desire and achieve the purpose for which I sent it."*[20] As I commit myself to you daily, I will become more mature in my walk and be strengthened to trust You in all things. In Jesus' name I pray, Amen.

Inner Tension

Let's Read from Genesis Chapter 25:19-34.

Jacob and Esau

This is the account of the family line of Abraham's son Isaac.

Abraham became the father of Isaac, and Isaac was forty years old when he married Rebekah daughter of Bethuel the Aramean from Paddan Aram and sister of Laban the Aramean.

Isaac prayed to the LORD on behalf of his wife, because she was childless. The LORD answered his prayer, and his wife Rebekah became pregnant. The babies jostled each other within her, and she said, "Why is this happening to me?" So she went to inquire of the LORD.

The LORD said to her,

> *"Two nations are in your womb,*
>> *and two peoples from within you will be separated;*
> *one people will be stronger than the other,*
>> *and the older will serve the younger."*

When the time came for her to give birth, there were twin boys in her womb. The first to come out was red, and his whole body was like a hairy garment; so they named him Esau. After this, his brother came out, with his hand grasping Esau's heel; so he was named Jacob. Isaac was sixty years old when Rebekah gave birth to them.

The boys grew up, and Esau became a skillful hunter, a man of the open country, while Jacob was content to stay at home among the tents. Isaac, who had a taste for wild game, loved Esau, but Rebekah loved Jacob.

Once when Jacob was cooking some stew, Esau came in from the open country, famished. He said to Jacob, "Quick, let me have some of that red stew! I'm famished!" (That is why he was also called Edom.)

Jacob replied, "First sell me your birthright."

"Look, I am about to die," Esau said. "What good is the birthright to me?"

But Jacob said, "Swear to me first." So he swore an oath to him, selling his birthright to Jacob.

Then Jacob gave Esau some bread and some lentil stew. He ate and drank, and then got up and left.

So Esau despised his birthright.

In Lesson 1, we discovered how an uncontrolled, undisciplined appetite lost mankind the crown to rule the earth and created broken fellowship with our Creator. Thousands of years later, many of the consequences of our "Super Size Me" culture's out-of-control appetites continue to be overlooked and ignored.

Appetites are very powerful. The ability (or inability) to manage them determines our direction in life. Perhaps someone you know handles their appetites quite well, and this is reflected in the way they live.

But for others, the deepest pain we experience in life can be the effect of the way someone else managed their appetites. Alcoholism, for example, has an effect on the alcoholic, as well as the family of the alcoholic.

A few essentials truths about appetites:

- **God created appetites, but sin distorted them.**
  Every single appetite you have has been broken, distorted, and corrupted by our sin nature.

- **Appetites are never fully satisfied.**
  Adam and Eve believed the lie that there was something else that could fully satisfy, but only God can meet all our needs.

- **Appetites always want it now!**
  Instead of waiting, we will trade (or forsake) something important for something immediate.

Esau was a man's-man and beloved by his father; Jacob was a momma's boy. They were twins; they were different; and Esau was born first, which caused conflict within the family.

The eldest son's special position was widely recognized in the ancient East. The privileges, highly valued, included a larger inheritance, family leadership, a place of honor at mealtime, and the paternal blessing (Genesis 25:5-6, 27:35-36, 37:21, 42:37, 43:33).

There were a few exceptions to the rule: Privileges could be forfeited by committing a serious offense (Genesis 35:22, 49:4), by paternal preference (Genesis 48:17), or by selling the privilege, as we see illustrated in the story of Jacob and Esau.

On the topic of Esau's priorities, The *Forerunner Commentary* states:

> He treasured his time out in the wild, and he had dedicated his life to pursuing the chase. By treasuring this "wild" existence over his birthright, Esau displayed how irresponsible he was toward it.
>
> Would we want to bequeath our wealth to a child who was not preparing himself to govern it? It would be similar to the prodigal son taking his inheritance and squandering it (Luke 15:11-13). He, like Esau, was not disciplined and trained to govern it. If most of Esau's time was spent out in the wild, how would he have been able to tackle the responsibilities of governing flocks and herds, gold and silver, male and female servants, donkeys and camels, as well as being his family's head and leader?[21]

We read that after having been out in the open country all day, Esau came to his younger brother Jacob and asked for some of his stew. The *Forerunner Commentary*, once again, offers great insight on what transpired that day:

His flesh was doing all the "thinking," as we see in his response to Jacob's opening offer: "And Esau said, 'Behold I am going to die; and what good is this birthright to me?'" (verse 32). Was he really so famished that he was going to die? Would he have said this had he been more involved with his inheritance and working with it?

If he had taken just a moment to think about his inheritance and what was involved, he would never have made such a rash decision. This could not have been the only food in the camp of a very wealthy man like Isaac; it was merely the first food he came to. Esau, the favorite of his father, could easily have gone to his father and told him what Jacob had tried to do and received food to satisfy his hunger. But he did not want to wait — he wanted immediate gratification of his fleshly desires.[22]

Thousands of studies in print and online explain how our brains respond to hunger. In essence, when any specific appetite becomes exaggerated, our brain magnifies it out of proportion. In response to this urge our brain signals that this food, this experience, or this person is going to be extraordinarily satisfying. What happens next is what we today call "buyer's remorse" or a sense of regret.

Our thinking changes when our appetites are provoked. Out-of-control appetites deliberately focus our thoughts on one thing and blur out everything else. Our attention then turns to that one food, one person, or one experience.

For **just one** bowl of lentil stew, Esau ultimately forfeited a larger inheritance, leadership of the family, the place of honor at the dinner table, Isaac's paternal blessing . . . and the blessing of Almighty God.

Hebrews 12:16-17 tells us:

> See that no one is sexually immoral, or is godless like Esau, who for a single meal sold his inheritance rights as the oldest son. Afterward, as you know, when he wanted to inherit this blessing, he was rejected. Even though he sought the blessing with tears, he could not change what he had done.

Who on earth would trade away their future for something so small?

We would.

We would do the same thing if it were the *right bowl of stew, soup, ice cream, etc.* For as long as we live in the flesh, this inner tension will exist and we will always be tempted to trade our future for something.

How do we ease this inner tension? Spiritual Discipline.

In surrenderring to Christ's power, we can *discipline* our minds to refrain from what we are about to do (which is sin) and master our thoughts. Paul pleads with us to *take captive every thought to make it obedient to Christ.*[23] He, himself, knew the power wielded by fleshly appetites and stated, *"I beat my body and make it my slave so that . . . I myself will not be disqualified for the prize."*[24] Our self-gratifying culture says we have the right to do and eat whatever and however we want. Our self-indulgent society says that we are the masters of our fate, and a pill, a diet program, or a diet-related surgical procedure will solve our sinful eating habits. This sentiment is captured in the last stanza of the Victorian poem, *Invictus*, by humanist William Earnest Hensley:

> It matters not how strait the gate,
> How charged with punishments the scroll.
> I am the master of my fate:
> I am the captain of my soul.[25]

On this subject, the Holy Spirit spoke through Paul when he wrote *"I have the right to do anything," you say — but not everything is beneficial. "I have the right to do anything" — but I will not be mastered by anything.*[26]

Look at your proverbial bowl of stew and ask yourself, "Is any type of food really worth it? Is it worth trading my future, my health, my relationships for immediate — and passing — gratification?"

The Lord Himself exhorted the ultimate solution to Adam and Eve's firstborn, Cain: *Sin is crouching at your door; it desires to have you, but you must master it.*[27]

What was true from the beginning is true for us today: Godly discipline is a vital ingredient to our freedom in Christ.

No discipline seems pleasant at the time, but painful. Later on, however, it produces a harvest of righteousness and peace for those who have been trained by it.

Hebrews 12:11

We end this lesson with the last stanza from Dorothea Day's poem, *My Captain*, her faith-based, Christian response to Hensley's *Invictus*.

> I have no fear, though strait the gate,
> He cleared from punishment the scroll.
> Christ is the Master of my fate,
> Christ is the Captain of my soul.

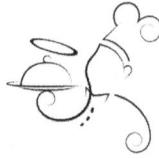

Mise en Place

Lose Sin – Gain Christ!

*Prayer/Devotion • Attitude • Hospitality • **Discipline** • Perseverance • Accountability*

Out-of-control eating and gluttony are, perhaps, the world's most unacknowledged sin. The prophets and apostles preached against it; yet we commonly engage in it. In general, Christians do not even recognize that when they overindulge, they're sinning.

To renew your mind, fill your soul with God's Word on the subject. Dig into the scriptures listed below and note answers in the space provided.

1) **Proverbs 21:20:** What is in the house of the wise? What does a foolish man/woman do?

   _____

   _____

2) **Proverbs 23:1-3:** What should we do if we are given to gluttony or overeating?

   _____

   _____

3) **Proverbs 23:6-8:** What food should we not eat? Why do you think this would be the case?

   _____

   _____

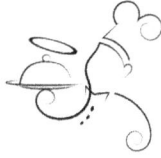

4) **Proverbs 23:21:** What happens to people who are gluttons?

_____

_____

5) **Romans 14:2-4:** What should be our attitude toward the way other people eat?

_____

_____

6) **John 6:27:** What type of food does Jesus tell us we should not work for? What type of food should we work for?

_____

_____

7) **Psalm 104:26-28:** Can the Lord satisfy your needs and desires as they relate to food?

_____

_____

Esau's Legacy Lentil Stew

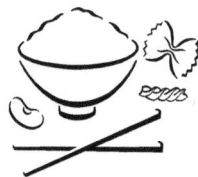

"Quick, let me have some of the red stew!
I'm famished!"

Genesis 25:30

Dating as far back at 6,000 B.C., lentils are one of the oldest cultivated crops. Lentils come in a variety of colors including green, brown, red, and yellow. You can purchase them dried or canned (preferrably dried.) Unlike other dried beans, lentils don't have to soak for hours before being cooked.

Sweet butternut squash, earthly lentils and a touch of roasted ground coriander are the winning combination in this homemade vegetarian stew. Esau may have given away his inheritance, but he most certainly would have prospered from the rich vitamins A and C, beneficial proteins, complex carbohydrates and filling fiber that pack this stew with goodness.

Ingredients

For all recipes contained in this study, God's Kitchen Ministries encourages the use of Certified Organic/Raw foods to maximize nutrition and gain the most health benefits.

- 2 tablespoons olive oil
- 1 cup chopped onions
- ½ cup carrots, cut into small cubes
- ½ cup celery, cut into small cubes
- 10 ounces butternut squash, cut into small cubes
- 1 pound lentils, picked and rinsed
- 14 ounce can diced tomatoes, drained
- 2 quarts (8 cups) chicken or vegetable broth
- 2 teaspoons roasted ground coriander (must be roasted)
- ½ teaspoon ground cumin
- ½ teaspoon each, kosher salt and ground black pepper, combined
- 1 tablespoon fresh parsley, finely chopped
- Greek yogurt, sour cream or crème fraiche to garnish

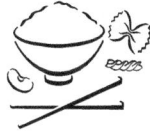

Instructions

Heat the olive oil in a large (6-quart) Dutch oven or heavy pot with a tight fitting lid. When the oil is hot, add the onions, carrots, celery, and butternut squash. Sweat for approximately 6-7 minutes until the onions are translucent. (To *sweat* is to cook, usually covered, in a small amount of fat over low heat. This method allows the food to soften without browning, and retains the natural juices.)

Add the lentils, drained tomatoes, broth, coriander, cumin, salt and ground pepper, and stir to combine. Increase the heat to high and bring to a boil. Once boiling, reduce the heat to low, cover and cook at a low simmer until the lentils are tender. This should take approximately 40 minutes.

Serve immediately "country-style" (in a serving dish from which everyone helps themselves), or puree in a blender to preferred consistency first.

Garnish servings with a teaspoon of yogurt, sour cream or crème fraiche and a touch of parsley.

Yield: About 6-8 cups. (Serving size: 1 cup)

For recipe photo and nutritional information, visit www.Gods-Kitchen.org.

Notes

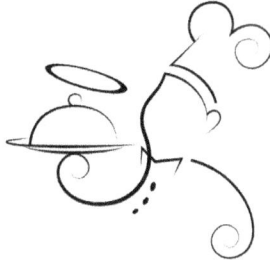

MULTI-COLORED TEMPTATIONS AND GRACE

Part I: First Course

Wherein ye greatly rejoice, though now for a season,
if need be, ye are in heaviness through manifold temptations.

1 Peter 1:6 KJV

In his first New Testament letter, the Apostle Peter wrote many words of encouragement to believers going through various forms of trials. He knew what he was talking about. During his lifetime, Peter experienced innumerable, multi-faceted temptations and trials of his own. (See Matthew 26:34, 69-75, Acts 4:1-20, Acts 5:17-42.) Through these life challenges, Peter discovered the Lord's immeasurable solution to his struggle with sin: The gift of God's manifold grace. *As every man hath received the gift, even so minister the same one to another, as good stewards of the manifold grace of God.* (1 Peter 4:10 KJV)

What is Grace?

Grace is the unmerited favor of God. It is something that is God-given, made possible only through the blood of Jesus Christ and none other. It is God's gift granted to sinners for their salvation.[28]

Our trials and temptations come in a wide spectrum of colors, and our Creator provides manifold shades of His Grace to match each one. As Paul wrote:

> *No temptation has seized you except what is common to man. And God is faithful; He will not let you be tempted beyond what you can bear. But when you are tempted, He will also provide a way out so that you can stand up under it.*
>
> 1 Corinthians 10:13

The implication is clear: God provides a way of escape for each particular trial and temptation we face. In the Book of Genesis, we find a vibrant illustration of this in the account of Joseph.

The story of Joseph — one of the twelve sons of Jacob — is my favorite story in the Bible, especially the powerful symbolism behind the famed multi-colored coat he received as a gift from his beloved father. It should be no surprise that this amazing gift would also symbolize the manifold trials he would experience in his lifetime, accompanied by God's manifold grace for each trial.

With the exception of Abraham, the history of Joseph takes up more space than any other narrative in the Old Testament. Because all scripture is God-breathed,[29] the Lord tells us, *"The Words I speak . . . will not return to me without producing results. They will accomplish what I want them to. They will do exactly what I sent them to do."*[30]

Joseph's life story presents us with countless scriptural precepts to learn, and reveal another ingredient for our Recipe for a Healthy and Holy Hunger: *Perseverance.*

To ensure optimum retention of each principle, we will take "smaller bites" and divide our study of Joseph into a "three-course meal."

Joseph's response to trials and temptations demonstrates how we can persevere in the face of our own enticements.

Let's begin today's lesson in prayful reverence — heads bowed and hearts exposed . . . .

Lord, You know the temptations that I face today, but your Word promises that I will not be tempted beyond what I can bear. I ask for your strength to stand up under the temptation whenever I encounter it. Your Word also tells me You will provide a way out of the temptation. Please, Lord, give me the wisdom to walk away when I am tempted and the clarity to see the way out that You will provide. Thank you, God, that you are a faithful deliverer and that I can count on your help in my time of need. In Christ Jesus' name I pray, Amen.

A Coat and a Dream

Let's read from Genesis, Chapter 37.

Joseph's Dreams

Jacob lived in the land where his father had stayed, the land of Canaan.

This is the account of Jacob's family line.

Joseph, a young man of seventeen, was tending the flocks with his brothers, the sons of Bilhah and the sons of Zilpah, his father's wives, and he brought their father a bad report about them.

Now Israel loved Joseph more than any of his other sons, because he had been born to him in his old age; and he made an ornate robe for him. When his brothers saw that their father loved him more than any of them, they hated him and could not speak a kind word to him.

Joseph had a dream, and when he told it to his brothers, they hated him all the more. He said to them, "Listen to this dream I had: We were binding sheaves of grain out in the field when suddenly my sheaf rose and stood upright, while your sheaves gathered around mine and bowed down to it."

His brothers said to him, "Do you intend to reign over us? Will you actually rule us?" And they hated him all the more because of his dream and what he had said.

Then he had another dream, and he told it to his brothers. "Listen," he said, "I had another dream, and this time the sun and moon and eleven stars were bowing down to me."

When he told his father as well as his brothers, his father rebuked him and said, "What is this dream you had? Will your mother and I and your brothers actually come and bow down to the ground before you?" His brothers were jealous of him, but his father kept the matter in mind.

Joseph Sold by His Brothers

Now his brothers had gone to graze their father's flocks near Shechem, and Israel said to Joseph, "As you know, your brothers are grazing the flocks near Shechem. Come, I am going to send you to them."

"Very well," he replied.

So he said to him, "Go and see if all is well with your brothers and with the flocks, and bring word back to me." Then he sent him off from the Valley of Hebron. . . .

So Joseph went after his brothers and found them near Dothan. But they saw him in the distance, and before he reached them, they plotted to kill him.

"Here comes that dreamer!" they said to each other. "Come now, let's kill him and throw him into one of these cisterns and say that a ferocious animal devoured him. Then we'll see what comes of his dreams."

When Reuben heard this, he tried to rescue him from their hands. "Let's not take his life," he said. "Don't shed any blood. Throw him into this cistern here in the wilderness, but don't lay a hand on him." Reuben said this to rescue him from them and take him back to his father.

So when Joseph came to his brothers, they stripped him of his robe — the ornate robe he was wearing — and they took him and threw him into the cistern. The cistern was empty; there was no water in it.

As they sat down to eat their meal, they looked up and saw a caravan of Ishmaelites coming from Gilead. Their camels were loaded with spices, balm and myrrh, and they were on their way to take them down to Egypt.

Judah said to his brothers, "What will we gain if we kill our brother and cover up his blood? Come, let's sell him to the Ishmaelites and not lay our hands on him; after all, he is our brother, our own flesh and blood." His brothers agreed.

So when the Midianite merchants came by, his brothers pulled Joseph up out of the cistern and sold him for twenty shekels of silver to the Ishmaelites, who took him to Egypt.

When Reuben returned to the cistern and saw that Joseph was not there, he tore his clothes. He went back to his brothers and said, "The boy isn't there! Where can I turn now?"

Then they got Joseph's robe, slaughtered a goat and dipped the robe in the blood. They took the ornate robe back to their father and said, "We found this. Examine it to see whether it is your son's robe."

He recognized it and said, "It is my son's robe! Some ferocious animal has devoured him. Joseph has surely been torn to pieces."

Then Jacob tore his clothes, put on sackcloth and mourned for his son many days. All his sons and daughters came to comfort him, but he refused to be comforted. "No," he said, "I will continue to mourn until I join my son in the grave." So his father wept for him.

Meanwhile, the Midianites sold Joseph in Egypt to Potiphar, one of Pharaoh's officials, the captain of the guard.

At the beginning of Chapter 37, Joseph, a teenager, had just literally "ratted on" his older brothers to their father. Consequently, Jacob's favoritism toward Joseph — demonstrated by the extravagant ornamental robe he gave Joseph — created vehement jealousy and hatred among his brothers.

In ancient times, a robe was a symbol of power and leadership. First Samuel 18:3-4 shows us evidence of this symbolism in the way Jonathan, the son and heir to King Saul, abdicated the kingship of Israel and transferred it to David: *Jonathan made a covenant with David because he loved him as himself. Jonathan took off the robe he was wearing and gave it to David, along with his tunic, and even his sword, his bow and his belt.*

After Joseph accepted the multi-colored "mantle of power" bestowed upon him by his beloved father, he had two divine dreams that symbolized how he would reign over his entire family. Genesis 37:8 tells us his brothers *hated him all the more because of his dreams and what he had said.*

Now, your first inclination may be to feel sympathy for his brothers, but they were by no means innocent; their true colors shone through as they plotted to kill — yes, kill — their little brother. By the Lord's providential hand, Joseph's brothers spared his life and then sold him to the Midianite traveling traders.

Let's read from Genesis 39 to see what happened next.

Joseph and Potiphar's Wife

The LORD was with Joseph so that he prospered, and he lived in the house of his Egyptian master. When his master saw that the LORD was with him and that the LORD gave him success in everything he did, Joseph found favor in his eyes and became his attendant. Potiphar put him in charge of his household and he entrusted to his care everything he owned. From the time he put him in charge of his household and of all that he owned, the LORD blessed the household of the Egyptian because of Joseph. The blessing of the LORD was on everything Potiphar had, both in the house and in the field. So Potiphar left everything he had in Joseph's care; with Joseph in charge, he did not concern himself with anything except the food he ate.

Now Joseph was well-built and handsome, and after a while his master's wife took notice of Joseph and said, "Come to bed with me!"

But he refused. "With me in charge," he told her, "my master does not concern himself with anything in the house; everything he owns he has entrusted to my care. No one is greater in this house than I am. My master has withheld nothing from me except you, because you are his wife. How then could I do such a wicked thing and sin against God?" And though she spoke to Joseph day after day, he refused to go to bed with her or even be with her.

One day he went into the house to attend to his duties, and none of the household servants were inside. She caught him by his cloak and said, "Come to bed with me!" But he left his cloak in her hand and ran out of the house. . . .

She kept his cloak beside her until his master came home. Then she told him this story: "That Hebrew slave you brought us came to me to make sport of me. But as soon as I screamed for help, he left his cloak beside me and ran out of the house."

When his master heard the story his wife told him, saying, "This is how your slave treated me," he burned with anger. Joseph's master took him and put him in prison, the place where the king's prisoners were confined.

But while Joseph was there in the prison, the LORD was with him; he showed him kindness and granted him favor in the eyes of the prison warden. So the warden put Joseph in charge of all those held in the prison, and he was made responsible for all that was done there. The warden paid *no attention to anything under Joseph's care, because the LORD was with Joseph and gave him success in whatever he did.*

For seventeen years, Joseph had been the apple of his father's eye and his "heir apparent." However, in the blink of an eye Joseph's life changed and his dreams appeared to become irrelevant. He was *sold as a slave. They bruised his feet with shackles, his neck was put in irons.*[31]

What types of temptations did Joseph face in bondage?

- to become sour on the world
    "Why do I try to do right? It doesn't pay! I'm now a slave and humiliated."

- to become sullen and bitter about his situation
    "Why did God let this happen to me?

Joseph had no control over his circumstances, but he knew Who was in control of his life — the God of Abraham, Isaac, and Jacob. Joseph never lost his faith and trust in God Almighty. Growing up, Joseph would have learned about Jacob's own life experiences and how God had provided. He would have known that Jacob had been forced to leave home (Genesis 28) and that God had been with him.

Joseph accepted his situation and adjusted to life as it was — even though it was not what he would have wished it to be, and definitely not what he had expected. He obediently worked as a slave, not because he was compelled to, but because he trusted God was with him (Genesis 39:2). He knew that the person who honors God will be blessed by God (Genesis 39:3-6).

Life took a turn for the better for Joseph (Genesis 39:1-6). Potiphar, the man who had bought Joseph, was one of Pharaoh's top officials. As captain of the guard he held a position equivalent to being the head of the Secret Service for the President of the United States. Potiphar noticed that Joseph's God *gave him success in everything he did,*[32] so, Potiphar put Joseph in charge of the entire household.

Think about that a moment. Potiphar handed over the entire running of his estate to Joseph. And because of Joseph, God blessed everything Potiphar had in his house and in his fields. Notice that the blessings were food-related! Scripture even tells us that after turning everything over to Joseph, Potiphar's only concern became the food set before him at meals.

As we look further into God's plan for Joseph, we will see more food-centric elements that reveal the Lord's "big picture" purpose.

What were Joseph's temptations in going from slave to the prosperity afforded him as personal steward?

- to forget God because all his physical needs were met

How did Joseph overcome this temptation?

- He was thankful to God for his prosperity, and saw the providential hand of God in his promotion.

As we know, though, success can be short-lived. Let's examine the attempted seduction of Joseph by Mrs. Potiphar (Genesis 39:7-20).

Joseph faced what temptations with Potiphar's wife?

- the flesh, and a 17-year old's adolescent hormones
- the desire for companionship — he was a long way from his home and his people
- taking the easy way out — submitting to her persistent advances. Who would ever know?

Of special note in the context of this story is the fact that Joseph lost another robe. The first cloak was taken away by his brothers. Mrs. Potiphar removed the second; she held it in her hands as Joseph escaped out the door. Two robes — symbols of power and authority — literally stripped from him.

How did Joseph persevere?

He recognized

- the sinfulness of her proposal — as sin against God, sin against Potiphar, sin against her, and sin against himself
- the value of character (self respect)

- his attitudes and actions were the seeds that would produce good fruit as he grew in both spirit and stature

There is something else of importance here, a principle that is of great value to us today. Joseph refused to be alone with this woman (Genesis 39:10).

Thousands of years before Ephesians 4:27 was ever written, Joseph made up his mind that he would not give the devil a foothold. He knew the best response to temptation is to RUN the opposite direction! However, when circumstances require us to submit to God's authority and stand our ground, the enemy will flee: *Submit yourselves, then, to God. Resist the devil, and he will flee from you. Come near to God, and he will come near to you* (James 4:7)

When Satan used food to deceive Eve into sinning, her response to his question (Genesis 3:1-2) revealed that she knew exactly what God had said.

Do we do likewise? When we know precisely what the Word of God says, do we often fail to obey Him?

We are now learning what God's Word says about eating. The question remains the same: Will we obey Him?

Do we spend more time indulging our appetites and desires than we do meditating on Scripture and praying? The enemy is relentless. His intention is to alienate humanity from our Creator, to stunt our growth as believers in Christ, and to minimize our service for God's Kingdom. He knows all our weakness (including our favorite foods that tempt us). That's why it is imperative to maintain a strong defense through an intimate, daily relationship with Jesus Christ. HE is our refuge, and His Word is a very effective weapon.

> *When you are tempted, you shouldn't say, "God is tempting me." God can't be tempted by evil. And he doesn't tempt anyone. But your own evil longings tempt you. They lead you on and drag you away. When they are allowed to grow, they give birth to sin. When sin has grown up, it gives birth to death.*
>
> James 1: 13-15

The Lord is holy; Satan is evil. God's Word teaches us to react to temptation with the understanding that its source is an evil enemy who *prowls around looking for someone to chew up and swallow* (1 Peter 5:8).

"Devil's food" is not chocolate; it's human souls. However, if we devour Holy Scripture, the devil will go hungry! King David knew God's truth when he wrote, *I have hidden your word in my heart that I might not sin against you* (Psalm 119:11).

Notes

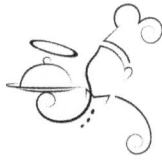

Mise en Place

Lose Sin – Gain Christ!

*Prayer/Devotion • Attitude • Hospitality • Discipline • **Perseverance** • Accountability*

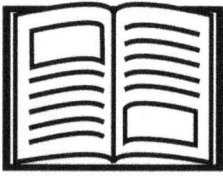

You have continued to work very faithfully these past few weeks and should be proud of your progress in committing to grow in your faith and please God with how you handle His provisions and blessings.

This week's Mise en Place is to start keeping a journal of the foods you consume and to document all temptations that come your way.

The point of the journal is not to track calories or points, but to get a realistic understanding of your eating habits, your food choices, your strengths, and your weaknesses.

Above all, I encourage you to be honest! The goal is to get a week's worth of insight into your current eating habits. Please do not omit foods because you want the journal to look "perfect." The only way to correct a problem is to identify its source so you can "Lose Sin" and "Gain Christ."

GOD'S KITCHEN

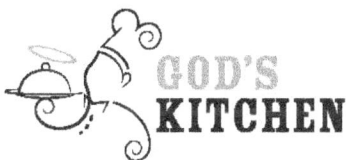

DAILY FOOD JOURNAL
For A Healthy & Holy Hunger

Day 1	What Did You Eat & Drink?	Hunger Level	Attitudes & Emotions	Temptations
Morning		Before Meal 0 1 2 3 4 5 After Meal 0 1 2 3 4 5		
Afternoon		Before Meal 0 1 2 3 4 5 After Meal 0 1 2 3 4 5		
Evening		Before Meal 0 1 2 3 4 5 After Meal 0 1 2 3 4 5		
Snack		Before Meal 0 1 2 3 4 5 After Meal 0 1 2 3 4 5		

Notes: _____

_____

_____

_____

_____

_____

_____

_____

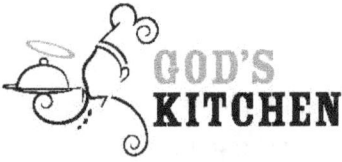

Day 2	What Did You Eat & Drink?	Hunger Level	Attitudes & Emotions	Temptations
Morning		Before Meal 0 1 2 3 4 5 After Meal 0 1 2 3 4 5	☹ ☹ 😐 🙂 😃	
Afternoon		Before Meal 0 1 2 3 4 5 After Meal 0 1 2 3 4 5	☹ ☹ 😐 🙂 😃	
Evening		Before Meal 0 1 2 3 4 5 After Meal 0 1 2 3 4 5	☹ ☹ 😐 🙂 😃	
Snack		Before Meal 0 1 2 3 4 5 After Meal 0 1 2 3 4 5	☹ ☹ 😐 🙂 😃	

Notes: _____

_____

_____

_____

_____

_____

_____

_____

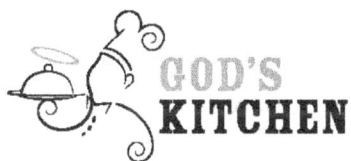

GOD'S KITCHEN

DAILY FOOD JOURNAL
For A Healthy & Holy Hunger

Day 3	What Did You Eat & Drink?	Hunger Level	Attitudes & Emotions	Temptations
Morning		Before Meal 0 1 2 3 4 5 After Meal 0 1 2 3 4 5	☹ ☹ 😐 ☺ 😀	
Afternoon		Before Meal 0 1 2 3 4 5 After Meal 0 1 2 3 4 5	☹ ☹ 😐 ☺ 😀	
Evening		Before Meal 0 1 2 3 4 5 After Meal 0 1 2 3 4 5	☹ ☹ 😐 ☺ 😀	
Snack		Before Meal 0 1 2 3 4 5 After Meal 0 1 2 3 4 5	☹ ☹ 😐 ☺ 😀	

Notes: _____

_____

_____

_____

_____

_____

_____

_____

GOD'S KITCHEN

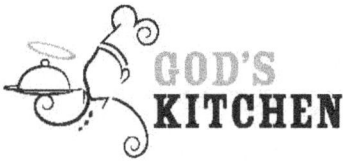

Lesson 5
DAILY FOOD JOURNAL
For A Healthy & Holy Hunger

Day 4	What Did You Eat & Drink?	Hunger Level	Attitudes & Emotions	Temptations
Morning		Before Meal 0 1 2 3 4 5 After Meal 0 1 2 3 4 5	☹ ☹ 😐 ☺ 😃	
Afternoon		Before Meal 0 1 2 3 4 5 After Meal 0 1 2 3 4 5	☹ ☹ 😐 ☺ 😃	
Evening		Before Meal 0 1 2 3 4 5 After Meal 0 1 2 3 4 5	☹ ☹ 😐 ☺ 😃	
Snack		Before Meal 0 1 2 3 4 5 After Meal 0 1 2 3 4 5	☹ ☹ 😐 ☺ 😃	

Notes: _____

_____

_____

_____

_____

_____

_____

_____

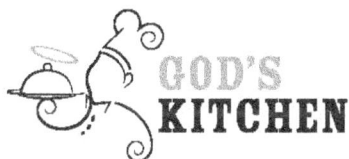

GOD'S KITCHEN

Day 5	What Did You Eat & Drink?	Hunger Level	Attitudes & Emotions	Temptations
Morning		Before Meal 0 1 2 3 4 5 After Meal 0 1 2 3 4 5	☹ ☹ 😐 ☺ 😃	
Afternoon		Before Meal 0 1 2 3 4 5 After Meal 0 1 2 3 4 5	☹ ☹ 😐 ☺ 😃	
Evening		Before Meal 0 1 2 3 4 5 After Meal 0 1 2 3 4 5	☹ ☹ 😐 ☺ 😃	
Snack		Before Meal 0 1 2 3 4 5 After Meal 0 1 2 3 4 5	☹ ☹ 😐 ☺ 😃	

Notes: _____

_____

_____

_____

_____

_____

_____

_____

GOD'S KITCHEN

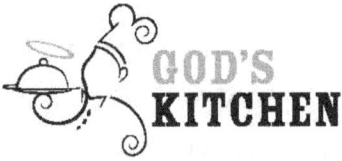

DAILY FOOD JOURNAL
For A Healthy & Holy Hunger

Day 6	What Did You Eat & Drink?	Hunger Level	Attitudes & Emotions	Temptations
Morning		Before Meal 0 1 2 3 4 5 After Meal 0 1 2 3 4 5	😖 😧 😐 😊 😃	
Afternoon		Before Meal 0 1 2 3 4 5 After Meal 0 1 2 3 4 5	😖 😧 😐 😊 😃	
Evening		Before Meal 0 1 2 3 4 5 After Meal 0 1 2 3 4 5	😖 😧 😐 😊 😃	
Snack		Before Meal 0 1 2 3 4 5 After Meal 0 1 2 3 4 5	😖 😧 😐 😊 😃	

Notes: _____

_____

_____

_____

_____

_____

_____

_____

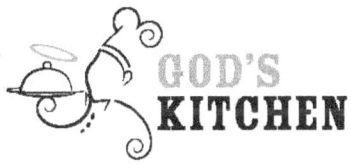

GOD'S KITCHEN

DAILY FOOD JOURNAL
For A Healthy & Holy Hunger

Day 7	What Did You Eat & Drink?	Hunger Level	Attitudes & Emotions	Temptations
Morning		Before Meal 0 1 2 3 4 5 After Meal 0 1 2 3 4 5	☹ ☹ 😐 ☺ 😃	
Afternoon		Before Meal 0 1 2 3 4 5 After Meal 0 1 2 3 4 5	☹ ☹ 😐 ☺ 😃	
Evening		Before Meal 0 1 2 3 4 5 After Meal 0 1 2 3 4 5	☹ ☹ 😐 ☺ 😃	
Snack		Before Meal 0 1 2 3 4 5 After Meal 0 1 2 3 4 5	☹ ☹ 😐 ☺ 😃	

Notes: _____

_____

_____

_____

_____

_____

_____

_____

Egyptian Pistachio Couscous with Roasted Chicken

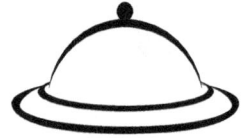

He did not concern himself with anything except the food that he ate.

Genesis 39:6

Joseph's leaving "in haste" made me think that we needed a quick and easy weeknight dinner recipe. The result was this "Cluck-of-the-Nile," lemony and nutty couscous dish. It was such a huge hit with the first God's Kitchen study group that everyone went home and made it for their mummies!

Ingredients

For all recipes contained in this study, God's Kitchen Ministries encourages the use of Certified Organic/Raw foods to maximize nutrition and gain the most health benefits.

- 2 tablespoons olive oil
- 2 cups chicken or vegetable stock
- 1 box Near East Couscous, Original Flavor (or equivalent)
- 1 grated lemon rind
- 3 ounces raisins
- 3 ounces pistachio nuts
- 2 ounces roasted almonds, sliced
- ½ teaspoon salt
- ½ teaspoon freshly ground black pepper
- 1 large, roasted chicken breast, chopped
- fresh flat-leaf parsley for garnish (optional)
- Recommended seasonings to taste: ground coriander, ground cumin, turmeric

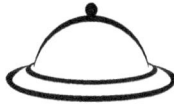

Instructions

Bring the stock and olive oil to boil in a medium saucepan.

Stir in the couscous; remove from the heat and cover. Allow to stand for 5 minutes.

Fluff couscous lightly with fork. Add the lemon rind, raisins, pistachio nuts and sliced, roasted almonds along with the salt and pepper.

To serve, place the couscous in a large bowl and arrange the chicken breast chucks over the top.

Pour the Lemon Vinaigrette* over couscous and chicken. Toss well to allow the flavors to mingle. Add additional seasonings to taste. Garnish with parsley.

*Lemon Vinaigrette

Ingredients

- ½ cup extra virgin olive oil
- 1 small shallot, minced or finely chopped
- 3 tablespoons fresh lemon juice
- 1 teaspoon lemon zest
- Salt and freshly ground black pepper

Instructions

Whisk the olive oil, shallot, lemon juice, lemon zest, salt and pepper until oil and juice become emulsified (combined).

Yield: 4 servings

For recipe photo and nutritional information, visit www.Gods-Kitchen.org.

Notes

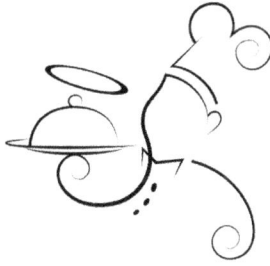

MULTI-COLORED TEMPTATIONS AND GRACE

Part II: Second Course

Potiphar left everything he had in Joseph's care; with Joseph in charge,
he did not concern himself with anything except the food he ate.

Genesis 39:6

As we learned in the previous lesson, in biblical times a robe, or cloak, was a sign of power, authority, and leadership. With leadership comes *Accountability*, our final ingredient in our Recipe for a Healthy and Holy Hunger.

Now let's consume the second course of this study on the life of Joseph in order to understand how to be accountable, as well as *more than conquerors*[33] in the face of temptation.

Temptation is something even Jesus experienced during His ministry here on earth. His disciples witnessed His victories, and took note of His unwavering prayer life. *"Teach us how to pray,"* the disciples said to Him (Luke 11:1). He answered by teaching them The Lord's Prayer. Although some tend to memorize this prayer as a set formula, its purpose was and is to awaken and stimulate our faith. Through this prayer, Jesus invites us to approach the God Most High, the All-Sufficient One who provides our daily bread, heals our infirmities and sanctifies us through and through. So it seems fitting to begin this lesson with that prayer:

> Father, hallowed be your name. Your kingdom come, your will be done, on earth as it is in heaven. Give us each day our daily bread. Forgive us our sins, for we also forgive everyone who sins against us. And lead us not into temptation, but deliver us from evil. For the kingdom, the power and the glory are yours. Now and forever, Amen. (Luke 11:2-4)

All I Have to Do Is Dream, Dream, Dream!

Let's Read from Genesis, Chapters 40 and 41.

Chapter 40:1-23

The Cupbearer and the Baker

Some time later . . . . Pharaoh was angry with his two officials, the chief cupbearer and the chief baker, and put them in custody in the house of the captain of the guard, in the same prison where Joseph was confined. The captain of the guard assigned them to Joseph, and he attended them.

After they had been in custody for some time, each of the two men . . . had a dream the same night, and each dream had a meaning of its own.

When Joseph came to them the next morning, he saw that they were dejected. So he asked . . . "Why do you look so sad today?"

"We both had dreams," they answered, "but there is no one to interpret them."

Then Joseph said to them, "Do not interpretations belong to God? Tell me your dreams."

So the chief cupbearer told Joseph his dream . . ."I saw a vine in front of me, and on the vine were three branches. As soon as it budded, it blossomed, and its clusters ripened into grapes. Pharaoh's cup was in my hand, and I took the grapes, squeezed them into Pharaoh's cup and put the cup in his hand."

"This is what it means," Joseph said to him. "The three branches are three days. Within three days Pharaoh will lift up your head and restore you to your position, and you will put Pharaoh's cup in his hand, just as you used to do when you were his cupbearer. But when all goes well with you,

remember me and show me kindness; mention me to Pharaoh and get me out of this prison. I was forcibly carried off from the land of the Hebrews, and even here I have done nothing to deserve being put in a dungeon."

When the chief baker saw that Joseph had given a favorable interpretation, he said to Joseph, "I too had a dream: On my head were three baskets of bread. In the top basket were all kinds of baked goods for Pharaoh, but the birds were eating them out of the basket on my head."

"This is what it means," Joseph said. "The three baskets are three days. Within three days Pharaoh will lift off your head and impale your body on a pole. And the birds will eat away your flesh."

Now the third day was Pharaoh's birthday, and he gave a feast for all his officials. . . . He restored the chief cupbearer to his position, so that he once again put the cup into Pharaoh's hand — but he impaled the chief baker, just as Joseph had said to them in his interpretation.

The chief cupbearer, however, did not remember Joseph; he forgot him.

We see in the recounting of the cupbearer and the baker that Joseph knew that God had not abandoned him. Both men asked him to interpret their dreams. His reply: *"Do not interpretations belong to God? Tell me your dreams"* (Genesis 40:8).

Having foreknowledge that the chief cupbearer would be restored to his prominent position in Pharaoh's court, Joseph sensed God's divine intervention in the situation and told the cupbearer his life story in hope that after he was reinstated the cupbearer would tell Joseph's story to Pharaoh. Upon his release from prison, the chief cupbearer did regain his title and fortune; however, he forgot about Joseph.

Do we treat God this way? If we are honest, the answer is *yes*. Typically, when the going gets tough, our anxious prayers are plentiful, but when the crisis is over and our comfort level returns, our urgent desire for prayer dissipates.

Once again, Joseph endured being ill-treated. The first time had been by his brothers; the second had been by Mrs. Potipher. Now, the third time, it was by the chief cupbearer.

Joseph had asked the cupbearer to work for his release. Though Joseph showed godly character in the Egyptian prison by not becoming angry and bitter in his heart, he still wanted his freedom, and used appropriate means to attempt to gain it. He thought the cupbearer's kindness might aid in prompt release from prison, but it was not to be. God had other plans.

Where did Joseph's strength to endure difficulties come from? We get a glimpse of his confidence and his mindset from verse 8: *Do not interpretations belong to God?* Joseph had personal experience with dreams. His two dreams about his future greatness had antagonized his brothers (Genesis 37:5-11), who mocked him (Genesis 37:19-20). Nevertheless, Joseph was confident that God would interpret these two men's dreams.

If Joseph was so confident about his fellow prisoners' dreams, might we assume he was confident that, someday, the Lord would bring his own two dreams to fruition?

Genesis Chapter 41

Pharaoh's Dreams

When two full years had passed, Pharaoh had a dream: He was standing by the Nile, when out of the river there came up seven cows, sleek and fat, and they grazed among the reeds. After them, seven other cows, ugly and gaunt, came up out of the Nile and stood beside those on the riverbank. And the cows that were ugly and gaunt ate up the seven sleek, fat cows. Then Pharaoh woke up.

He fell asleep again and had a second dream: Seven heads of grain, healthy and good, were growing on a single stalk. After them, seven other heads of grain sprouted — thin and scorched by the east wind. The thin heads of grain swallowed up the seven healthy, full heads. . . .

In the morning his mind was troubled, so he sent for all the magicians and wise men of Egypt. Pharaoh told them his dreams, but no one could interpret them for him.

Then the chief cupbearer said to Pharaoh, "Today I am reminded of my shortcomings. Pharaoh was once angry with his servants, and he imprisoned me and the chief baker in the house of the captain of the guard. Each of us had a dream the same night, and each dream had a meaning of its own. Now a young Hebrew was there with us, a servant of the captain of the guard. We told him our dreams, and he interpreted them for us, giving each man the interpretation of his dream. And things turned out exactly as he interpreted them to us: I was restored to my position, and the other man was impaled."

So Pharaoh sent for Joseph, and he was quickly brought from the dungeon. When he had shaved and changed his clothes, he came before Pharaoh.

Pharaoh said to Joseph, "I had a dream, and no one can interpret it. But I have heard it said of you that when you hear a dream you can interpret it."

"I cannot do it," Joseph replied to Pharaoh, "but God will give Pharaoh the answer he desires." . . .

"God has shown Pharaoh what he is about to do. Seven years of great abundance are coming throughout the land of Egypt, but seven years of famine will follow them. Then all the abundance in Egypt will be forgotten, and the famine will ravage the land. The abundance in the land will not be remembered, because the famine that follows it will be so severe. The reason the dream was given to Pharaoh in two forms is that the matter has been firmly decided by God, and God will do it soon.

"And now let Pharaoh look for a discerning and wise man and put him in charge of the land of Egypt. Let Pharaoh appoint commissioners over the land to take a fifth of the harvest of Egypt during the seven years of abundance. They should collect all the food of these good years that are coming and store up the grain under the authority of Pharaoh, to be kept in the cities for food. This food should be held in reserve for the country, to be used during the seven years of famine that will come upon Egypt, so that the country may not be ruined by the famine." . . . .

Then Pharaoh said to Joseph, "Since God has made all this known to you, there is no one so discerning and wise as you. You shall be in charge of my palace, and all my people are to submit to your orders. Only with respect to the throne will I be greater than you."

Joseph in Charge of Egypt

So Pharaoh said to Joseph, "I hereby put you in charge of the whole land of Egypt." Then Pharaoh took his signet ring from his finger and put it on Joseph's finger. He dressed him in robes of fine linen and put a gold chain around his neck. He had him ride in a chariot as his second-in-command and people shouted before him, "Make way!" Thus he put him in charge of the whole land of Egypt.

Then Pharaoh said to Joseph, "I am Pharaoh, but without your word no one will lift hand or foot in all Egypt."...

Joseph was thirty years old when he entered the service of Pharaoh king of Egypt. And Joseph went out from Pharaoh's presence and traveled throughout Egypt. During the seven years of abundance the land produced plentifully. Joseph collected all the food produced in those seven years of abundance in Egypt and stored it in the cities. In each city he put the food grown in the fields surrounding it. Joseph stored up huge quantities of grain, like the sand of the sea; it was so much that he stopped keeping records because it was beyond measure. . . .

The seven years of abundance in Egypt came to an end, and the seven years of famine began, just as Joseph had said. . . . And all the world came to Egypt to buy grain from Joseph, because the famine was severe everywhere.

For thirteen years, the Lord shaped and molded Joseph by putting him in positions to be a steward in Potiphar's household, and later, manager of the prison ward. Joseph was then ready to interpret Pharaohs dreams, be put in charge of the whole land of Egypt, and ultimately save God's people from famine and death.

Have you noticed how the story of Joseph centers on God providing food for His people? Blessings and provisions of food abounded because of Joseph's character and his accountability to those he served and to the Lord. God will take care of your needs in this area, too, if you will be accountable with what He gives you!

Do you recall the two coats taken from Joseph? The first, removed and ruined by his own brothers. The second, removed by Potiphar's wife. But the third robe became a Judicial Robe![34] With it, Joseph acquired more power and influence than he ever dreamed.

Isn't that like our God to go beyond our wildest dreams and expectations? Paul put it succinctly in Ephesians 3:20:

Now to Him who is able to do immeasurably more than all we ask or imagine, according to His power that is at work within us, to Him be glory in the church and in Christ Jesus throughout all generations, for ever and ever! Amen.

"Throughout all generations" refers to us.

What would happen if we handed over our sinful eating habits to God?

Notes

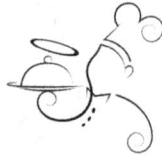

Mise en Place

Lose Sin – Gain Christ!

*Prayer/Devotion • Attitude • Hospitality • Discipline • **Perseverance** • Accountability*

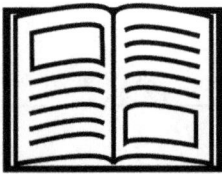

This week's Mise en Place is to continue recording in your journal the foods you consume during the week, and to document all temptations that come your way.

In addition to tracking eating habits, attitudes and temptations, you will also invite the Lord into your daily dining!

Each day select a Scripture verse about food that is meaningful to you. Choose from any one of the verses found in the previous lessons, or from those you researched in the Mise En Place assignments. Write the verse at the top of the page each morning before you have breakfast.

As you add to your journal throughout the day, God's love will be your guide and strengthen your commitment to acquire a Healthy and Holy Hunger.

In Proverbs 3:2-4, Solomon instructed each of us to take God's words and do the following:

Bind them around your neck,

write them on the tablet of your heart.

Then you will win favor and a good name

in the sight of God and man.

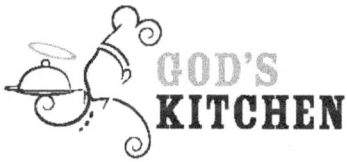

GOD'S
KITCHEN

DAILY FOOD JOURNAL
For A Healthy & Holy Hunger

Scripture Verse Of The Day

Day 1	What Did You Eat & Drink?	Hunger Level	Attitudes & Emotions	Temptations
Morning		Before Meal 0 1 2 3 4 5 After Meal 0 1 2 3 4 5	☹ 🙁 😐 🙂 😃	
Afternoon		Before Meal 0 1 2 3 4 5 After Meal 0 1 2 3 4 5	☹ 🙁 😐 🙂 😃	
Evening		Before Meal 0 1 2 3 4 5 After Meal 0 1 2 3 4 5	☹ 🙁 😐 🙂 😃	
Snack		Before Meal 0 1 2 3 4 5 After Meal 0 1 2 3 4 5	☹ 🙁 😐 🙂 😃	

Notes: _____
_____
_____
_____
_____

GOD'S KITCHEN

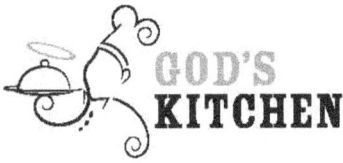

DAILY FOOD JOURNAL
For A Healthy & Holy Hunger

Scripture Verse Of The Day

Day 2	What Did You Eat & Drink?	Hunger Level	Attitudes & Emotions	Temptations
Morning		Before Meal 0 1 2 3 4 5 After Meal 0 1 2 3 4 5	☹ ☹ 😐 ☺ 😃	
Afternoon		Before Meal 0 1 2 3 4 5 After Meal 0 1 2 3 4 5	☹ ☹ 😐 ☺ 😃	
Evening		Before Meal 0 1 2 3 4 5 After Meal 0 1 2 3 4 5	☹ ☹ 😐 ☺ 😃	
Snack		Before Meal 0 1 2 3 4 5 After Meal 0 1 2 3 4 5	☹ ☹ 😐 ☺ 😃	

Notes: _____
_____
_____
_____
_____

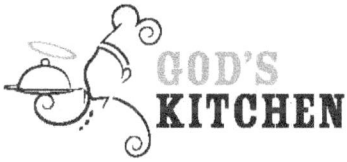

GOD'S KITCHEN

Lesson 6
DAILY FOOD JOURNAL
For A Healthy & Holy Hunger

Scripture Verse Of The Day

Day 3	What Did You Eat & Drink?	Hunger Level	Attitudes & Emotions	Temptations
Morning		Before Meal 0 1 2 3 4 5 After Meal 0 1 2 3 4 5	☹ ☹ 😐 ☺ 😃	
Afternoon		Before Meal 0 1 2 3 4 5 After Meal 0 1 2 3 4 5	☹ ☹ 😐 ☺ 😃	
Evening		Before Meal 0 1 2 3 4 5 After Meal 0 1 2 3 4 5	☹ ☹ 😐 ☺ 😃	
Snack		Before Meal 0 1 2 3 4 5 After Meal 0 1 2 3 4 5	☹ ☹ 😐 ☺ 😃	

Notes: _____

_____

_____

_____

_____

GOD'S KITCHEN

Lesson 6

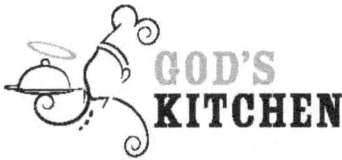

DAILY FOOD JOURNAL
For A Healthy & Holy Hunger

Scripture Verse Of The Day

Day 4	What Did You Eat & Drink?	Hunger Level	Attitudes & Emotions	Temptations
Morning		Before Meal 0 1 2 3 4 5 / After Meal 0 1 2 3 4 5	☹ ☹ 😐 ☺ 😀	
Afternoon		Before Meal 0 1 2 3 4 5 / After Meal 0 1 2 3 4 5	☹ ☹ 😐 ☺ 😀	
Evening		Before Meal 0 1 2 3 4 5 / After Meal 0 1 2 3 4 5	☹ ☹ 😐 ☺ 😀	
Snack		Before Meal 0 1 2 3 4 5 / After Meal 0 1 2 3 4 5	☹ ☹ 😐 ☺ 😀	

Notes: _____
_____
_____
_____
_____

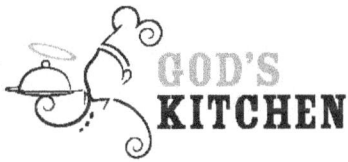

GOD'S KITCHEN

DAILY FOOD JOURNAL
For A Healthy & Holy Hunger

Scripture Verse Of The Day

Day 5	What Did You Eat & Drink?	Hunger Level	Attitudes & Emotions	Temptations
Morning		Before Meal 0 1 2 3 4 5 After Meal 0 1 2 3 4 5	☹ ☹ 😐 🙂 😃	
Afternoon		Before Meal 0 1 2 3 4 5 After Meal 0 1 2 3 4 5	☹ ☹ 😐 🙂 😃	
Evening		Before Meal 0 1 2 3 4 5 After Meal 0 1 2 3 4 5	☹ ☹ 😐 🙂 😃	
Snack		Before Meal 0 1 2 3 4 5 After Meal 0 1 2 3 4 5	☹ ☹ 😐 🙂 😃	

Notes: _____

_____

_____

_____

_____

GOD'S KITCHEN

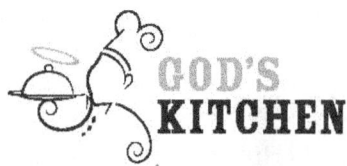

Lesson 6
DAILY FOOD JOURNAL
For A Healthy & Holy Hunger

Scripture Verse Of The Day

Day 6	What Did You Eat & Drink?	Hunger Level	Attitudes & Emotions	Temptations
Morning		Before Meal 0 1 2 3 4 5 After Meal 0 1 2 3 4 5	☹ ☹ ☺ ☺ ☺	
Afternoon		Before Meal 0 1 2 3 4 5 After Meal 0 1 2 3 4 5	☹ ☹ ☺ ☺ ☺	
Evening		Before Meal 0 1 2 3 4 5 After Meal 0 1 2 3 4 5	☹ ☹ ☺ ☺ ☺	
Snack		Before Meal 0 1 2 3 4 5 After Meal 0 1 2 3 4 5	☹ ☹ ☺ ☺ ☺	

Notes: _____
_____
_____
_____
_____

GOD'S KITCHEN

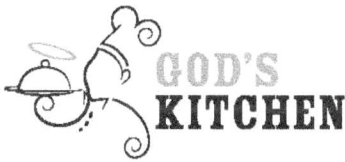

Lesson 6
DAILY FOOD JOURNAL
For A Healthy & Holy Hunger

Scripture Verse Of The Day

Day 7	What Did You Eat & Drink?	Hunger Level	Attitudes & Emotions	Temptations
Morning		Before Meal 0 1 2 3 4 5 After Meal 0 1 2 3 4 5	☹ ☹ 😐 ☺ 😀	
Afternoon		Before Meal 0 1 2 3 4 5 After Meal 0 1 2 3 4 5	☹ ☹ 😐 ☺ 😀	
Evening		Before Meal 0 1 2 3 4 5 After Meal 0 1 2 3 4 5	☹ ☹ 😐 ☺ 😀	
Snack		Before Meal 0 1 2 3 4 5 After Meal 0 1 2 3 4 5	☹ ☹ 😐 ☺ 😀	

Notes: _____
_____
_____
_____
_____

Pharoah's Fat and Lean Black and White All-Purpose Cake

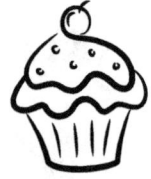

Pharaoh had a dream. . . .

Genesis 41:1

This all-purpose, black and white cake is a dream come true. You only need one bowl and one whisk to make it, so there's less clean up required in the kitchen! And it takes just 10 minutes to prepare. Perfect for breakfast, for dessert, or as a snack.

Ingredients

For all recipes contained in this study, God's Kitchen Ministries encourages the use of Certified Organic/Raw foods to maximize nutrition and gain the most health benefits.

- 6 tablespoons butter
- 1 cup sugar
- 1½ teaspoons vanilla extract
- 4 large egg whites
- ¾ cup low-fat buttermilk
- ½ teaspoon salt
- ½ teaspoon baking soda
- 1½ cups all-purpose flour
- 3 tablespoons unsweetened cocoa
- ¼ teaspoon almond extract
- nuts to taste (optional)

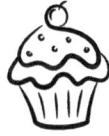

Instructions

Preheat oven to 350°.

Coat an 8-inch square baking pan with cooking spray and dust with flour.

Melt the butter over a low heat and mix together with the sugar in a large bowl. Add the vanilla and egg whites, whisking well. Stir in the buttermilk, salt, and baking soda.

Lightly spoon the flour into dry measuring cups and level with a knife. Add to the mixture, stirring gently until just blended. Be careful not to overstir the batter once the flour is added, or the flour's gluten will be activated and toughen the cake's texture.

Spread half of the batter into the prepared pan. Gently stir the cocoa and almond extract into the remaining batter. If you wish to add nuts, stir them in at the last minute.

Slowly layer the chocolate batter over the batter in the pan.

Bake for 30 minutes or until a wooden pick inserted into the center comes out clean.

Cool for 10 minutes in the pan on a wire rack. Cut into squares. Top with powdered sugar or fruit.

Yield: 9 servings (Serving size: 1 slice)

For recipe photo and nutritional information, visit www.Gods-Kitchen.org.

Notes

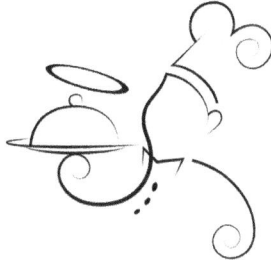

Multi-Colored Temptations and Grace

Part III: Third Course

The Boys Are Back In Town

What would you do with unlimited power?

Such was Joseph's position.

The famine had created an international disaster. People from surrounding nations heard that only Egypt had enough provisions to survive the famine ravaging their world.

Who should arrive to buy grain but Joseph's brothers, the same brothers who had thrown him into a pit to starve while they ate their lunch oblivious to his cries for help.

Having endured the suffering, injustice, and neglect sparked by the actions of his brothers, Joseph now faced possibly his greatest test of character.

Can you imagine the thoughts that went through Joseph's mind? His brothers were destitute and defenseless in this land. He had unlimited power, and the opportunity to use it against them.

It is one thing to resist temptation when you are powerless. It is quite another to resist when you have the opportunity to exact revenge because your enemies are at your mercy.

While poverty, suffering, and injustice are trials that can come our way, like Joseph, we are usually tested most by what we are given and the way that we use it. God-led self-control is the key.

The same principle applies to our approach to food. For this reason, we must take a hard look at what enabled Joseph to use the power at his disposal for the betterment of his brothers rather than as an opportunity to vent all the bitter feelings that could have been his.

Let's begin our final course with prayer.

> Father God, I realize there will be times when I am faced with temptations and life-altering choices. I pray that, through the leading of Your Holy Spirit, I will take to heart the example set before me through the amazing historical account of your servant, Joseph. Prayer time with You strengthens me against temptation, as your Word says in Mark 14:38: *Watch and pray so that you will not fall into temptation. The spirit is willing, but the flesh is weak.* You gave Joseph discernment and used him in a mighty way to feed and save others. In the name of Jesus Christ, my Savior, I ask You to do the same with me. Amen.

Let's read from Genesis, Chapters 42-45.

Chapter 42

Joseph's Brothers Go to Egypt

> *When Jacob learned that there was grain in Egypt, he said to his son. . . "Go down there and buy some for us, so that we may live and not die. . . ."*
>
> *But Jacob did not send Benjamin, Joseph's brother, with the others, because he was afraid that harm might come to him. . . .*
>
> *Now Joseph was the governor of the land, the person who sold grain to all its people. So when Joseph's brothers arrived, they bowed down to him with their faces to the ground. As soon as Joseph saw his brothers, he recognized them, but he pretended to be a stranger and spoke harshly to them. "Where do you come from?" he asked.*
>
> *"From the land of Canaan," they replied, "to buy food. . . ."*
>
> *Then he remembered his dreams about them and said to them, "You are spies! You have come to see where our land is unprotected."*

"No, my lord," they answered. "Your servants have come to buy food. . . . Your servants are honest men, not spies. . . .

"Your servants were twelve brothers, the sons of one man, who lives in the land of Canaan. The youngest is now with our father, and one is no more . . . ."

Joseph said to them . . . "This is how you will be tested. . . . Send one of your number to get your brother." . . . And he put them all in custody for three days.

On the third day, Joseph said to them . . . "Do this and you will live, for I fear God: If you are honest men, let one of your brothers stay here in prison, while the rest of you go and take grain back for your starving households. But you must bring your youngest brother to me, so that your words may be verified and that you may not die." This they proceeded to do. . . .

He had Simeon taken from them and bound before their eyes.

Joseph gave orders to fill their bags with grain, to put each man's silver back in his sack, and to give them provisions for their journey. After this was done for them, they loaded their grain on their donkeys and left.

At the place where they stopped for the night one of them opened his sack to get feed for his donkey, and he saw his silver in the mouth of his sack. . . .

Their hearts sank and they turned to each other trembling and said, "What is this that God has done to us?"

When they came to their father Jacob in the land of Canaan, they told him all that had happened to them. . . .

As they were emptying their sacks, there in each man's sack was his pouch of silver! When they and their father saw the money pouches, they were frightened. Their father Jacob said to them, "You have deprived me of my children. Joseph is no more and Simeon is no more, and now you want to take Benjamin. Everything is against me! . . .

"My son will not go down there with you; his brother is dead and he is the only one left. If harm comes to him on the journey you are taking, you will bring my gray head down to the grave in sorrow."

Genesis 43

The Second Journey to Egypt

Now the famine was still severe in the land. So when they had eaten all the grain they had brought from Egypt, their father said to them, "Go back and buy us a little more food."

But Judah said to him. . . . "If you will send our brother along with us, we will go down and buy food for you. But if you will not send him, we will not go down, because the man said to us, 'You will not see my face again unless your brother is with you.' . . ."

Their father Israel said to them . . . "If it must be . . . take your brother . . . and go back to the man at once. And may God Almighty grant you mercy before the man so that he will let your other brother and Benjamin come back with you. As for me, if I am bereaved, I am bereaved."

So the men took . . . gifts and double the amount of silver, and Benjamin also. They hurried down to Egypt and presented themselves to Joseph. When Joseph saw Benjamin with them, he said to the steward of his house, "Take these men to my house, slaughter an animal and prepare a meal; they are to eat with me at noon. . . ."

When Joseph came home, they presented to him the gifts they had brought into the house, and they bowed down before him to the ground. He asked them how they were, and then he said, "How is your aged father you told me about? Is he still living?"

They replied, "Your servant our father is still alive and well." And they bowed down, prostrating themselves before him.

As he looked about and saw his brother Benjamin, his own mother's son, he asked, "Is this your youngest brother, the one you told me about?" And he said, "God be gracious to you, my son." Deeply moved at the sight of his brother, Joseph hurried out and looked for a place to weep. He went into his private room and wept there.

After he had washed his face, he came out and . . . said, "Serve the food. . . . "

The men had been seated before him in the order of their ages, from the firstborn to the youngest; and they looked at each other in astonishment. When portions were served to them from Joseph's table, Benjamin's portion was five times as much as anyone else's. So they feasted and drank freely with him.

Genesis 44

A Silver Cup in a Sack

Now Joseph gave these instructions to the steward of his house: "Fill the men's sacks with as much food as they can carry, and put each man's silver in the mouth of his sack. Then put my cup, the silver one, in the mouth of the youngest one's sack, along with the silver for his grain." And he did as Joseph said.

As morning dawned, the men were sent on their way with their donkeys. They had not gone far from the city when Joseph said to his steward, "Go after those men at once, and when you catch up with them, say to them, 'Why have you repaid good with evil?'. . ."

When he caught up with them . . . they said to him, "Why does my lord say such things? . . . If any of your servants is found to have it, he will die; and the rest of us will become my lord's slaves. . . ."

Then the steward proceeded to search, beginning with the oldest and ending with the youngest. And the cup was found in Benjamin's sack. At this, they tore their clothes. Then they all loaded their donkeys and returned to the city.

Joseph was still in the house when Judah and his brothers came in, and they threw themselves to the ground before him. Joseph said to them, "What is this you have done?. . . The man who was found to have the cup will become my slave. The rest of you, go back to your father in peace."

Then Judah went up to him and said: "Pardon your servant, my lord, let me speak a word to my lord. Do not be angry with your servant, though you are equal to Pharaoh himself. . . . If the boy is not with us when I go back to your servant my father, and if my father, whose life is closely bound up with the boy's life, sees that the boy isn't there, he will die. . . . Your servant guaranteed the boy's safety to my father. . . . Now then, please let your servant remain here as my lord's slave in place of the boy, and let the boy return with his brothers. How can I go back to my father if the boy is not with me? No! Do not let me see the misery that would come on my father."

Genesis 45

Joseph Makes Himself Known

Then Joseph could no longer control himself before all his attendants, and he cried out, "Have everyone leave my presence!" So there was no one with Joseph when he made himself known to his brothers. . . .

Then Joseph said to his brothers, "Come close to me." When they had done so, he said, "I am your brother Joseph, the one you sold into Egypt! And now, do not be distressed and do not be angry with yourselves for selling me here, because it was to save lives that God sent me ahead of you. For two years now there has been famine in the land, and for the next five years there will be no plowing and reaping. But God sent me ahead of you to preserve for you a remnant on earth and to save your lives by a great deliverance.

"So then, it was not you who sent me here, but God. He made me father to Pharaoh, lord of his entire household and ruler of all Egypt. Now hurry back to my father and say to him, 'This is what your son Joseph says: God has made me lord of all Egypt. Come down to me; don't delay. You shall live in the region of Goshen and be near me — you, your children and grandchildren, your flocks and herds, and all you have. I will provide for you there, because five years of famine are still to come. Otherwise you and your household and all who belong to you will become destitute.'

"You can see for yourselves, and so can my brother Benjamin, that it is really I who am speaking to you. Tell my father about all the honor accorded me in Egypt and about everything you have seen. And bring my father down here quickly."

Then he threw his arms around his brother Benjamin and wept, and Benjamin embraced him, weeping. And he kissed all his brothers and wept over them. Afterward his brothers talked with him.

When the news reached Pharaoh's palace that Joseph's brothers had come, Pharaoh and all his officials were pleased. Pharaoh said to Joseph, "Tell your brothers, 'Do this: Load your animals and return to the land of Canaan, and bring your father and your families back to me. I will give you the best of the land of Egypt and you can enjoy the fat of the land.'

"You are also directed to tell them, 'Do this: Take some carts from Egypt for your children and your wives, and get your father and come. Never mind about your belongings, because the best of all Egypt will be yours.'"

So the sons of Israel did this. Joseph gave them carts, as Pharaoh had commanded, and he also gave them provisions for their journey. To each of them he gave new clothing, but to Benjamin he gave three hundred shekels of silver and five sets of clothes. And this is what he sent to his father: ten donkeys loaded with the best things of Egypt, and ten female donkeys loaded with grain and bread and other provisions for his journey. Then he sent his brothers away. . . .

So they went up out of Egypt and came to their father Jacob in the land of Canaan. They told him, "Joseph is still alive! In fact, he is ruler of all Egypt."

In order to appreciate Joseph's ability to resist temptation and be self-controlled, we must understand some biblical principles:

1. **Power is wrapped up in stewardship.** From the beginning of the creation, power was given to man by God:

   Then God said, "Let us make man in our image, according to our likeness; and let him rule over the fish of the sea and over the birds of the sky and over the cattle and over all the earth, and over every creeping thing that creeps on the earth.

   Genesis 1:26

   In Genesis 9:5-7, governing authority was given to man. This power is reaffirmed in the New Testament:

   Let every person be in subjection to the governing authorities, for there is no authority except from God, and those which exist are established by God.

   Romans 13:1

   When Pilate sought to evoke a response from Jesus by impressing Him with the authority he had, Jesus quickly put this power in proper perspective: It was delegated power, given by God.

   Jesus answered, "You would have no authority over Me, unless it had been given to you from above."

   John 19:11

   Joseph was well aware that God had given him any power he had. We can see this, for example, when Pharaoh told Joseph that he was aware of his ability to interpret dreams. Joseph was quick to clarify that this power was not his, but God's:

Pharaoh said to Joseph, "I have had a dream, but no one can interpret it; and I have heard it said about you, that when you hear a dream you can interpret it." Joseph then answered Pharaoh, saying, "It is not in me; God will give Pharaoh a favorable answer."

Genesis 41:15-16

The first step toward the misuse of our own willpower is to forget the source from which our power comes and to overlook the responsibility required of us as stewards.

2. Power has a purpose.

Even the Son of Man did not come to be served, but to serve, and to give His life a ransom for many.

Mark 10:45

As Joseph recalled his dreams, he must have realized that his power was God-given not to satisfy his own selfish desires, but to save the nation of Israel from physical famine. Therefore, he gave grain freely to his brothers rather than allowing them to starve.

3. Spiritual results come from spiritual power.

It might have been a great temptation for Joseph to get even with his brothers for the evil they had done to him. But Joseph employed his secular power to benefit his brothers. Still, it was his spiritual power that produced the greatest results. While Joseph's artificial harshness to his brothers produced fear, his graciousness resulted in spiritual awareness and the beginning of repentance.

His bothers also experienced "manifold grace" as they considered their circumstances as coming from the hand of God. It was only after Joseph released his brothers from prison and relaxed his demands and offered hope and life by assuring them that he, too, feared God (Genesis 42:18) that they began to consider God's hand in their dilemma (Genesis 42:21-22). Moreover, it was after they realized that their money was given back to them in the grain sack that they said, *"What is this that God has done to us?"* (Genesis 42:28).

How clear this all becomes in the light of the teaching of the Apostle Paul in the book of Romans:

Never pay back evil for evil to anyone. Respect what is right in the sight of all men. If possible, so far as it depends on you, be at peace with all men. Never take your own revenge, beloved, but leave room for the wrath of God, for it is written, "Vengeance is Mine, I will repay," says the Lord. "But if your enemy is hungry, feed him, and if he is thirsty, give him a drink; for in so doing you will heap burning coals upon his head." Do not be overcome by evil, but overcome evil with good.

Romans 12:17-21 NASB

That is what Joseph's dealings with his brothers were about. They were hungry and he fed them. He was in a position to unleash all of his feelings of anger and bitterness, but instead, he used the spiritual power of God, which he demonstrated by serving and setting the interests of others first.

This selfless spirit of Joseph is a remarkable contrast to the self-seeking spirit of Jacob and his ten sons. Spiritual power, exercised from godly motives, brings about spiritual ends.

The question the story of Joseph leaves us with is this: How do we exercise our willpower, especially as it relates to food? Do we use it to serve God, or to seek our own selfish ends?

In the beginning of this lesson, we discussed the manifold/multi-colored trials and temptations and how accountability to God and others is an irreplaceable component.

Joseph, the Apostles, and many other saints learned these precepts the same way you and I do — one day at a time. Each saw how God's manifold grace provided a precise way of escape for each temptation.

Whatever multi-colored trials we face — food or otherwise — the indescribable colors of God's Grace are sufficient for every trial you encounter, including the gastronomic.

We must all bear in mind that ultimately we are each accountable to God:

> *So then each of us shall give account of himself to God.*
>
> Romans 14:12
>
> *What will I do when God confronts me? What will I answer when called to account?*
>
> Job 31:14

Joseph had a firm grasp of this precept:

> *"How then can I do this great wickedness, and sin against God?"*
>
> Genesis 39:9

His reply needs to become a personal conviction for each of us in the face of temptation.

Acquiring a Healthy and Holy Hunger depends on developing our own personal relationship with God out of sincere love, fear, and reverence. It truly means to eat in a manner pleasing to Him. For biblical accountability to fulfill its purpose, we must come to this place.

Like Joseph, and like Jesus, we are to rely on the Lord and know that our manifold temptations and the testing our faith produce perseverance.

> *Let perseverance finish its work so that you may be mature and complete, not lacking anything.*
>
> James 1: 2-4

Notes

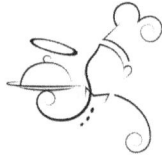

Mise en Place

Lose Sin - Gain Christ!

Prayer/Devotion • Attitude • Hospitality • Discipline • Perseverance • **Accountability**

BREAKING THE YOKE!

"Take my yoke upon you and learn from me, for I am gentle and humble in heart, and you will find rest for your souls. For my yoke is easy and my burden is light."
Matthew 11:29-30

We know our sins are a heavy yoke and a constant burden, but what makes Jesus' yoke easier and His burden lighter? His perfect obedience to the Father, and His decision to carry the burden we were meant to carry. For the believer, it is the indwelling Holy Spirit who has the power to bring change to our lives and mold us into the image of Christ.

Our final Mise en Place is the sweetest . . . and is served with humility.

The Apostle Paul told the Corinthians *the kingdom of God is not a matter of talk but of power* (1 Corinthians 4:20). The time has come to trade your weak willpower for God's willpower and allow Him to break the yoke of food's tyranny in your life! As with the last journal assignment, continue to prayerfully select a food-related verse daily and record the foods you consume and your hunger levels.

This week's new journal elements are to list any eating habit or attitude you altered — or temptation you resisted — through the power of the Holy Spirit and incorporate the Recipe for a Healthy and Holy Hunger ingredients of *Prayer, Devotion, Attitude, Hospitality, Discipline, Perseverance,* and *Accountability* into your daily routine.

What will be the result of this yoke-breaking culinary creation? Spirit-led changes to your eating habits, His desire will become your desire, and your kitchen will gradually become God's Kitchen. As our Master so eloquently put it: *"My food . . . is to do the will of Him who sent me and to finish His work"* (John 4:34).

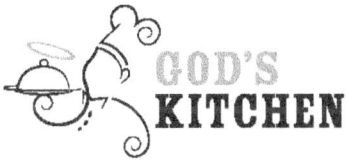

GOD'S KITCHEN

DAILY FOOD JOURNAL
For A Healthy & Holy Hunger

Scripture Verse Of The Day

Day 1	What Did You Eat & Drink?	Hunger Level	Broke A Yoke!	Holy Hunger Ingredients:
Morning		Before Meal 0 1 2 3 4 5 After Meal 0 1 2 3 4 5	*(List any eating habit or attitude you altered-or temptation you resisted-through the power of the Holy Spirit.)*	*(Circle all that applied today.)* *Prayer* *Devotion*
Afternoon		Before Meal 0 1 2 3 4 5 After Meal 0 1 2 3 4 5		*Attitude* *Hospitality*
Evening		Before Meal 0 1 2 3 4 5 After Meal 0 1 2 3 4 5		*Discipline* *Perseverance*
Snack		Before Meal 0 1 2 3 4 5 After Meal 0 1 2 3 4 5		*Accountability*

Notes: _____

_____

_____

_____

_____

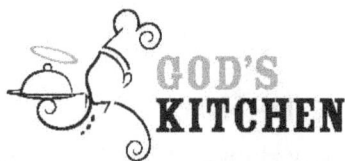

GOD'S KITCHEN

Lesson 7

DAILY FOOD JOURNAL
For A Healthy & Holy Hunger

Scripture Verse Of The Day

Day 2	What Did You Eat & Drink?	Hunger Level	Broke A Yoke!	Holy Hunger Ingredients:
Morning		Before Meal 0 1 2 3 4 5 After Meal 0 1 2 3 4 5	*(List any eating habit or attitude you altered-or temptation you resisted-through the power of the Holy Spirit.)*	*(Circle all that applied today.)* Prayer Devotion
Afternoon		Before Meal 0 1 2 3 4 5 After Meal 0 1 2 3 4 5		Attitude Hospitality
Evening		Before Meal 0 1 2 3 4 5 After Meal 0 1 2 3 4 5		Discipline Perseverance
Snack		Before Meal 0 1 2 3 4 5 After Meal 0 1 2 3 4 5		Accountability

Notes: _____
_____
_____
_____
_____

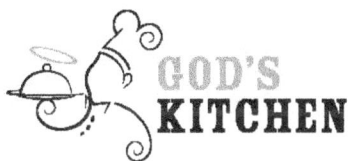

Scripture Verse Of The Day

Day 3	What Did You Eat & Drink?	Hunger Level	Broke A Yoke!	Holy Hunger Ingredients:
Morning		Before Meal 0 1 2 3 4 5 After Meal 0 1 2 3 4 5	*(List any eating habit or attitude you altered-or temptation you resisted-through the power of the Holy Spirit.)*	*(Circle all that applied today.)* *Prayer* *Devotion*
Afternoon		Before Meal 0 1 2 3 4 5 After Meal 0 1 2 3 4 5		*Attitude* *Hospitality*
Evening		Before Meal 0 1 2 3 4 5 After Meal 0 1 2 3 4 5		*Discipline* *Perseverance*
Snack		Before Meal 0 1 2 3 4 5 After Meal 0 1 2 3 4 5		*Accountability*

Notes: _____

_____

_____

_____

_____

GOD'S KITCHEN

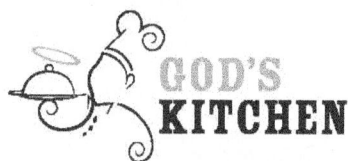

DAILY FOOD JOURNAL
For A Healthy & Holy Hunger

Scripture Verse Of The Day

Day 4	What Did You Eat & Drink?	Hunger Level	Broke A Yoke!	Holy Hunger Ingredients:
Morning		Before Meal 0 1 2 3 4 5 After Meal 0 1 2 3 4 5	*(List any eating habit or attitude you altered-or temptation you resisted-through the power of the Holy Spirit.)*	*(Circle all that applied today.)* *Prayer* *Devotion*
Afternoon		Before Meal 0 1 2 3 4 5 After Meal 0 1 2 3 4 5		*Attitude* *Hospitality*
Evening		Before Meal 0 1 2 3 4 5 After Meal 0 1 2 3 4 5		*Discipline* *Perseverance*
Snack		Before Meal 0 1 2 3 4 5 After Meal 0 1 2 3 4 5		*Accountability*

Notes: _____

_____

_____

_____

_____

GOD'S KITCHEN

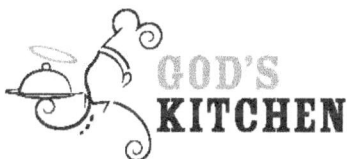

DAILY FOOD JOURNAL
For A Healthy & Holy Hunger

Day 5	What Did You Eat & Drink?	Hunger Level	Broke A Yoke!	Holy Hunger Ingredients:
Morning		Before Meal 0 1 2 3 4 5 After Meal 0 1 2 3 4 5	(List any eating habit or attitude you altered-or temptation you resisted-through the power of the Holy Spirit.)	(Circle all that applied today.) Prayer Devotion
Afternoon		Before Meal 0 1 2 3 4 5 After Meal 0 1 2 3 4 5		Attitude Hospitality
Evening		Before Meal 0 1 2 3 4 5 After Meal 0 1 2 3 4 5		Discipline Perseverance
Snack		Before Meal 0 1 2 3 4 5 After Meal 0 1 2 3 4 5		Accountability

Notes: _____
_____
_____
_____
_____

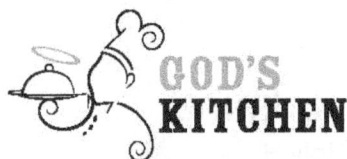

GOD'S KITCHEN

Lesson 7
DAILY FOOD JOURNAL
For A Healthy & Holy Hunger

Day 6	What Did You Eat & Drink?	Hunger Level	Broke A Yoke!	Holy Hunger Ingredients:
Morning		Before Meal 0 1 2 3 4 5 After Meal 0 1 2 3 4 5	*(List any eating habit or attitude you altered-or temptation you resisted-through the power of the Holy Spirit.)*	*(Circle all that applied today.)* *Prayer* *Devotion*
Afternoon		Before Meal 0 1 2 3 4 5 After Meal 0 1 2 3 4 5		*Attitude* *Hospitality*
Evening		Before Meal 0 1 2 3 4 5 After Meal 0 1 2 3 4 5		*Discipline* *Perseverance*
Snack		Before Meal 0 1 2 3 4 5 After Meal 0 1 2 3 4 5		*Accountability*

Notes: _____
_____
_____
_____
_____

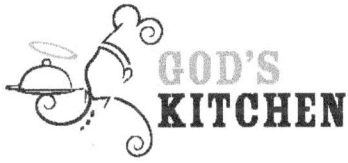

GOD'S KITCHEN

Lesson 7

DAILY FOOD JOURNAL

For A Healthy & Holy Hunger

Scripture Verse Of The Day

Day 7	What Did You Eat & Drink?	Hunger Level	Broke A Yoke!	Holy Hunger Ingredients:
Morning		Before Meal 0 1 2 3 4 5 After Meal 0 1 2 3 4 5	*(List any eating habit or attitude you altered-or temptation you resisted-through the power of the Holy Spirit.)*	*(Circle all that applied today.)* *Prayer* *Devotion*
Afternoon		Before Meal 0 1 2 3 4 5 After Meal 0 1 2 3 4 5		*Attitude* *Hospitality*
Evening		Before Meal 0 1 2 3 4 5 After Meal 0 1 2 3 4 5		*Discipline* *Perseverance*
Snack		Before Meal 0 1 2 3 4 5 After Meal 0 1 2 3 4 5		*Accountability*

Notes: _____
_____
_____
_____
_____

"Finally Free"-keh Pilaf

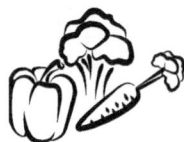

"I have heard that there is grain in Egypt.
Go down there and buy some for us, so that we may live and not die."

Genesis 42:2

An ancient Mediterranean superfood that is worth discovering, *freekeh* (also known as *farik* or *frika*) has been around for centuries. Freekeh is young wheat, harvested while still green, then smoked or roasted. It has *four times* the fiber of brown rice. The grains have a nutty "green tea" flavor and are quite filling. Combined with rich, savory veggies and dried fruits, it makes an exotic pilaf that is to die for! If you can't find freekeh locally, you can order it online.

Ingredients

For all recipes contained in this study, God's Kitchen Ministries encourages the use of Certified Organic/Raw foods to maximize nutrition and gain the most health benefits.

- 1 cup dry freekeh
- 1 teaspoon apple cider vinegar
- 1 small red onion, diced
- 1 tablespoon of butter
- 12 ounces of mushrooms, chopped
- extra virgin olive oil
- ½ teaspoon sea salt
- 2 cloves garlic, minced
- ¼ cup or less white wine or chicken stock (to deglaze the pan)
- ¼ cup pine nuts
- ½ cup chopped dried apricots
- salt and pepper to taste
- crumbled Feta cheese or goat cheese, to taste
- fresh chopped parsley, for garnish

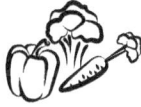

Instructions

Soak the freekeh in water and 1 teaspoon of apple cider vinegar overnight. (This helps to break up the phytic acid, which inhibits the absorption of all those amazing minerals in the freekeh.) Drain and rinse. Combine the freekeh with 1 cup of water in a saucepan. Bring it to a boil, then cover and cook on low heat until freekeh has absorbed all the water.

While the freekeh is cooking, cook the onion in butter over low heat until caramelized (richly browned). Add mushrooms, a small amount of olive oil (to prevent the butter from burning), and salt. Sauté for 5 minutes.

Add minced garlic to the onion-mushroom mixture. Cook until liquid has evaporated and mushrooms start to sear. Deglaze with the white wine or chicken stock. (Deglaze by adding the liquid to the pan and stirring until it reaches a boil. This loosens and dissolves the flavor-packed brown bits stuck to the bottom of the pan. Deglazing can make a flavorful sauce or gravy.)

Add the steamed freekeh, pine nuts, and chopped apricots to the onion-mushroom-garlic mixture. Stir to combine. Cook for additional 5 minutes. Add crumbled feta (or goat) cheese, then salt and pepper to taste.

Transfer the mixture to a bowl, garnish with fresh, chopped parsley and serve.

Note: In the U.S. freekeh can be purchased in specialty markets that carry natural or Middle Eastern foods.

Yield: 6-8 servings (Serving size: ½-⅔ cup)

For recipe photo and nutritional information, visit www.Gods-Kitchen.org.

Notes

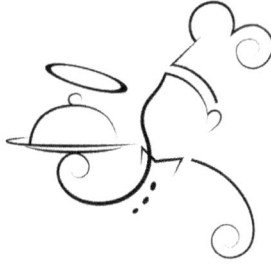

THE THIRD GARDEN: BREAKING THE YOKE

Stand fast therefore in the liberty by which Christ has made us free.

Galatians 5:1

The Garden Tomb

At the place where Jesus was crucified, there was a garden,
and in the garden a new tomb, in which no one had ever been laid.

John 19:4

The Lord Almighty's perfect and omniscient plan of salvation for mankind was planted, pruned, and the precious fruit plucked and harvested in three holy gardens: the Garden of Eden, the Garden of Gethsemane, and The Garden Tomb, which is the site of Jesus' burial and resurrection. An invitation to dine at God's table (for all eternity) was made possible through the Fall of Mankind, the Suffering of God's Anointed, and the Atonement of His Holy Blood.

The Garden Tomb is where Christ conquered sin, triumphed over death, and Satan was condemned.[35] Have you ever wondered what type of plants would have adorned this miraculous site? Jewish tradition tells us that crops, such as cabbages or lettuce, were grown here.[36] Scripture also tells us that there was a gardener employed there (Mary Magdalene thought the resurrected Jesus was the gardener[37]). But a gardener in first century Israel would not have been hired to simply care for flowers. Judging from other archeological findings of garden tombs from that period, historians believe that grapes, olives, and other vegetables may have been a part of the Garden Tomb site as well.

Just think: The greatest event in history — where our freedom was won and our slavery ended — took place in a garden that offered nourishment. Two life-giving sources of nourishment for all mankind to feed on that abundantly satisfy our spiritual and physical desires!

The yoke has been broken, my friend, so that we can experience a relationship with our Creator and enjoy — without guilt and shame — the provisions He gives us.

> *I am the LORD your God, who brought you out of Egypt so that you would no longer be slaves to the Egyptians; I broke the bars of your yoke and enabled you to walk with heads held high.*

Leviticus 26:13

Some terms in the Bible have multiple (and symbolic) meanings. The word *Egypt* not only represents the actual country, but also the act of sin.[38] Scripture tells us that God not only saved the Israelites from the land of Egypt, but also saved us from all our sins. Before God began working with us, we had no power over sin; we were slaves to it, just as the Israelites were literal slaves to the Egyptians. When we choose to follow God and His way of life, we no longer serve sin but God, and God gives us everlasting life. The apostle Paul wrote,

> *Formerly, when you did not know God, you were slaves to those who by nature are not gods. But now that you know God — or rather are known by God — how is it that you are turning back to those weak and miserable principles? Do you wish to be enslaved by them all over again?*

Galatians 4:8-9

Why do we continue to act like slaves when we have been freed from sin's hold through Christ's blood? If you have not yet made that decision, my friend, it is my prayer that you will do so today. Tell God that you want to become His child and a follower of His Son, Jesus Christ, and that you are ready to give Him control for the remainder of your life. Your prayer could go something like this . . .

Lord, there are too many cooks in my kitchen! I am sorry for trying to run my own life. I resign as of today. I believe your Son, Jesus Christ, paid my death penalty when He died on the cross. I'm turning from a life of "my way" and I'm putting all my trust in Jesus Christ, to give me a relationship with You and to welcome me into heaven. Lord, from today on, I am yours, Amen.

Remember, Jesus said,

> *"Greater love has no one than this, that he lay down his life for his friends. You are my friends if you do what I command. I no longer call you slaves, because a slave does not know his master's business. Instead, I have called you friends, for everything that I learned from my Father I have made known to you. You did not choose me, but I chose you and appointed you to go and bear fruit — fruit that will last."*

John 15:13-16

A lot of God's Word poured into you during this study. If you truly desire it, that can bring freedom and powerful change to your life — freedom from the yoke, the bondage, and the tyranny of harmful eating habits, as well as other idols and addictions you might be dealing with.

Remember the recipe of God's Kitchen that will strengthen and encourage you along the way:

Prayer/Devotion • Attitude • Hospitality • Discipline • Perseverance • Accountability

Now that you have tasted and seen how devouring Holy Scripture can help you overcome, I encourage you to continue consuming His Daily Bread because, as John 8:31 tells us, Jesus said, *"If you hold to my teaching, you are really my disciples. Then you will know the truth, and the truth will set you free."*

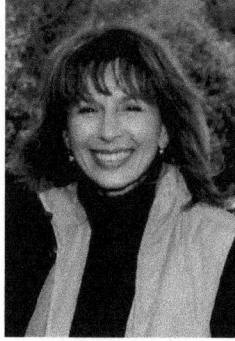

In Memoriam
MARIANN FERREIRA
1956 - 2012
Love God. Love People. Serve Both.

Mariann Ferreira walked the Christian's narrow path with enthusiasm, both spiritually and physically. She took great care of her "temple" by eating to please her Lord and Savior and by committing to daily, invigorating walks. She was renowned for sharing the Gospel — and all she had — with the lost.

Mariann hungered for God's Word and personified our ministry's purpose: to teach and encourage the surrendering of hearts and minds to the power of the Holy Spirit, who counsels and nourishes our bodies, our souls, and our spirits.

A victim of violent crime, Mariann walked through Heaven's Gates on December 2, 2012.

It was a privilege and an honor to befriend Mariann Ferreira, a great saint and warrior for God's Kingdom. To honor her legacy, we offer one of her signature dessert recipes.

Mariann's Homespun & Wholesome Rice Pudding

Ingredients

- 1 cup organic long grain rice
- water
- 7¾ cups whole (raw) milk
- 3 organic eggs, lightly beaten
- 1 cup raw honey
- 2 tablespoons natural vanilla extract
- cinnamon (to taste)
- nutmeg (to taste)

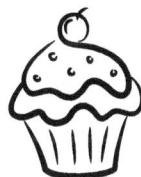

Instructions

Place rice in a large pot and add just enough water to cover it. Bring to a boil, then simmer until all water is absorbed. Add milk and simmer for 1 hour with the lid on the pot, stirring frequently so it does not stick to the bottom of the pot or boil over. Cool slightly.

Beat eggs, honey, and vanilla together in a large mixing bowl. To this egg mixture, add two or three ladles of the cooked rice — one and a time, stirring after each — to temper the eggs. Then, add the rest of the cooked rice and stir. Return the mixture to the pot and cook for 5 more minutes, stirring constantly. Place the mixture in a large serving bowl. Sprinkle with cinnamon and a dash of nutmeg.

Yield: 6 servings (Serving size: 1 cup)

For recipe photo and nutritional information, visit www.Gods-Kitchen.org.

ABOUT THE AUTHOR

Cook-for-Christ Toni Perry is an award-winning Bible study teacher, author, certified *cuisinière*, food educator, and inspirational speaker committed to educating believers to eat healthy, eat holy, and find comfort in God's provisions. Her God's Kitchen Ministries — www.gods-kitchen.org — focuses on teaching God's Word in a culinary classroom environment to encourage women to taste the truth about food and understand how eating and attitudes affect our relationship with God and others.

Toni and the God's Kitchen Ministries staff also serve their local Morris County, New Jersey community through a faith-based grief outreach by providing meals to those who are mourning the loss of a loved one.

Toni's lessons in Christ and cuisine began at the age of nine under the tutelage of her Italian grandmother who taught her to serve the Lord humbly through hospitality and the *arti culinarie*. After Toni obtained a Bachelor of Arts degree in foreign language study from Rutgers University, she became a perpetual student of cooking, in both the United States and abroad.

She currently holds a position as an Adjunct Professor of Hospitality Management and Culinary Arts at The County College of Morris in New Jersey and is a Certified Instructor for the National Restaurant Association Educational Foundation (NRAEF).

Toni combines her communication skills, biblical insight, and extensive collection of innovative recipes to offer an interactive, fun, and delectable way to study and learn the life-giving precepts and promises found in the Bible.

Throughout the years, trust and faith in Jesus Christ have brought Toni through many of life's "coarsely chopped" moments, including divorce, single parenting, a 10-year battle with cancer, and overcoming a lifelong struggle with food.

Toni and her husband, George, have a blended family of four adult children and two grandchildren. They reside in a quaint, lake-community bungalow in New Jersey.

ENDNOTES

1   Author Unknown

2   Genesis 3:20

3   merriam-webster.com

4   Matthew 26:36-46, Mark 14:32-51, and Luke 22:40-46

5   Guthrie. Nancy, *Jesus, Keep Me Near the Cross*: *Experiencing the Passion and Power of Easter*, Copyright 2009, (Wheaton, Illinois, Crossway Books), pp. 31-32.

6   Genesis 3:12

7   Genesis 3:13

8   Crabtree, Dr. David, *Answers to Chapter Two*, McKenzie Study Center, Copyright February 2002, internet article. http://msc.gutenberg.edu/2002/02/answers-to-chapter-two/

9   Ibid.

10 Fitzpatrick, Elyse, *Love to Eat, Hate to Eat: Breaking the Bondage of Destructive Eating Habits*, Copyright 1999, (Eugene, OR, Harvest House Publishers), pg. 102

11 Genesis 6:6

12 Genesis 6:5

13 Hebrews 11:7

14 Woodmorappe, John, 1996. *Noah's Ark: A Feasibility Study*. Santee, CA: Institute for Creation Research, pp. 153-162.

15 Mark 14:36, Romans 8:15, and Galatians 4:6

16 www.definitions.net/definition/hospitality

17 Bierce, Ambrose, *The Collected Words of Ambrose Bierce*, Volume IV, Shapes of Clay, (New York and Washington, The Neale Publishing Company,) Copyright 1910, pg. 357.

18 Ennis, Patricia, *Practicing Biblical Hospitality*, Journal for Biblical Manhood and Womanhood, (Santa Clarita, CA. Fall 2006 11/2), pp. 117-118.

19 Matthew 19:26 and Mark 10:27

20 Isaiah 55:11

21 Staff, Bibletools.org, Forerunner Commentary, *What Is Your Lentil Soup?* http://www.bibletools.org/index.cfm/fuseaction/Library.sr/CT/RA/k/1052

22 Ibid.

23 2 Corinthians 10:5

24 1 Corinthians 9:27

25 wikipedia.org/wiki/Invictus

26 1 Corinthians 6:12

27 Genesis 4:7

28 wikipedia.org/wiki/Divine_grace

29 2 Timothy 3:16

30 Isaiah 55:11

31 Psalm 105: 17-18

32 Genesis 39:3

33 Romans 8:37

34 Genesis 41:33

35 John 16:11

36 Price, Robert M., *Jesus' Burial In The Garden: The Strange Growth Of The Tradition*, RMP Theological Publications, Copyright 2006, http://www.robertmprice.mindvendor.com/burial.htm

37 John 20:15

38 www.bibletools.org, topic: Egypt-as-Sin, http://www.bibletools.org/index.cfm/fuseaction/Topical.show/RTD/cgg/ID/5943/Egypt-as-Sin.htm

www.ingramcontent.com/pod-product-compliance
Lightning Source LLC
Chambersburg PA
CBHW080517090426
42734CB00015B/3091